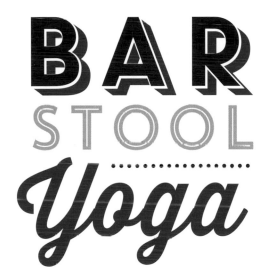

BAR STOOL Yoga

THE FUN
WAY OF
BEING FIT
AND
FLEXIBLE
AT THE
BAR
AND
BEYOND

• MIRIAM AUSTIN •

Photography by Stephen Hunter

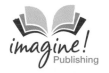

imagine!
Publishing

To my brother and best friend, Mike, who helped me behind the scenes in more ways than I can count. Without you this book would not have been nearly as fabulous as it is. I cannot thank you enough. You're the greatest! –MA

10 9 8 7 6 5 4 3 2 1

An Imagine Book
Published by Charlesbridge
85 Main Street
Watertown, MA 02472
617-926-0329
www.charlesbridge.com

Text copyright © 2014 Miriam Austin.
Interior and cover design by Melissa Gerber.
Photos copyright © 2014 Charlesbridge Publishing, Inc.
Back cover photo © Shutterstock/199483742/homydesign

Printed in China, October 2014.

ISBN: 978-1-62354-047-0

For information about custom editions, special sales, premium and corporate purchases, please contact Charlesbridge Publishing, Inc. at specialsales@charlesbridge.com.

CONTENTS

CAUTION

WE ABSOLUTELY, POSITIVELY DO NOT WANT ANYONE TO INJURE THEMSELVES BY DRINKING COCKTAILS, WINE, OR BEER AND DOING YOGA ON A BAR STOOL. THIS BOOK IS WHIMSICAL AND FUN, NOT A RECIPE FOR HOW YOGA SHOULD NORMALLY BE PRACTICED. PLEASE ENJOY YOUR WINE, BEER, OR COCKTAILS AFTER YOUR YOGA PRACTICE, NOT DURING IT.

Achieving balance in our modern world is not easy. Pressed for time, people have turned to yoga to fulfill their needs for physical fitness, relaxation, a deep spiritual life, and an active social life. Yoga has become both the coolest exercise and the coolest form of community. The yoga studio is where we exercise, release our stress, meet new people, and see old friends. We feel more relaxed, more energetic, and our worries (and pains in the neck) exit as we leave the yoga studio. We feel great in our bodies, so we feel great in our spirits. We then naturally want to connect with people in our community in a more meaningful way after class. We want to have fun, and what better way than having a beer, a glass of wine, dinner, or a cup of coffee together!?

Bar Stool Yoga takes this fun a little bit further. Our union is with other people. Our spiritual experience includes the distilled spirits in a convivial atmosphere. The bar stool becomes a favorite prop. Our favorite poses are renamed after some of the world's most famous drinks—or obscure drinks, in some cases.

Yogis and yoginis are often seen stretching in public places. Some airports now have yoga rooms. Corporations, parks, schools, churches, communities of all types all offer yoga classes. Why? Because yoga makes us feel so good. We feel exhilarated and we want to shout it from the rooftops. We want to convert everyone we know. So let's take yoga to the places it hasn't been yet: bars and restaurants. Do poses with your yoga friends. Show your non-yoga friends the cool tricks you have learned in yoga class. In essence, *Bar Stool Yoga* is about the sheer joy of yoga and sharing that joy with our friends—wherever we are.

And, one more thing: There are thousands of guys who have told their girls, "Sure, honey, I'll do yoga … when they start having classes at my local bar." Hey, guys, no more excuses.

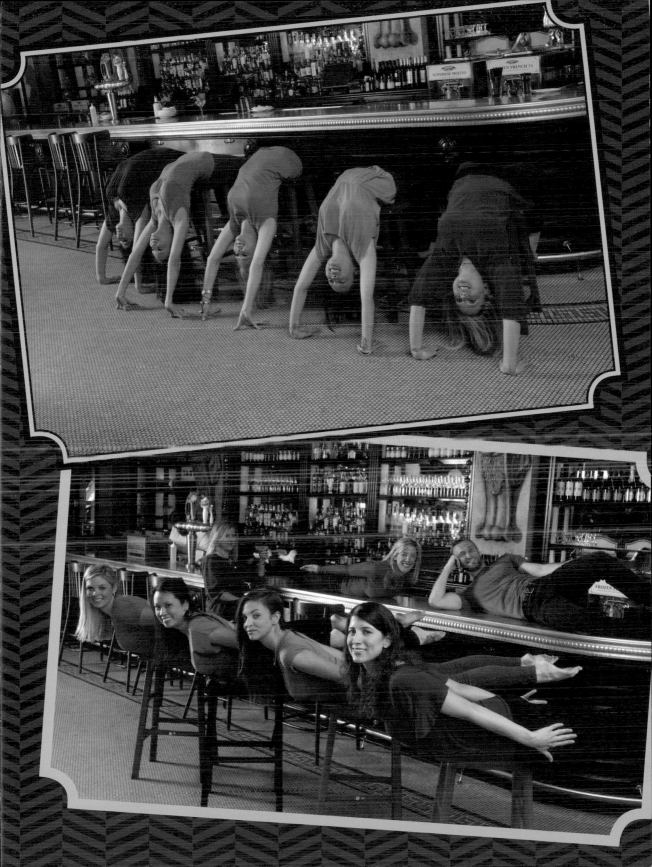

HOW TO PREPARE FOR BAR STOOL YOGA

Preparing for yoga in a bar is not much different from preparing for yoga in your home or at the studio. Anywhere you practice yoga, the first rule is safety. First, do no harm to yourself. So many of us want to go beyond our limits in yoga. We stretch too much or twist too deeply or attempt a pose we are not quite ready for. In our enthusiasm, we sometimes fail to warm up sufficiently. Other times we forget some of the basic alignment keys that protect our joints and muscles. And when we are not fully conscious of proper form and preparation, we pull a muscle, overstretch a ligament, or tweak our backs or necks. So always remember to prepare for poses.

Basic Stretching

Before any yoga practice, and particularly before attempting bar stool yoga, practice a few basic stretches. Stretch your arms, shoulders, legs, thighs, and calves. Then do a couple of fundamental poses, such as Downward Facing Dog, Lunge, and Plank. If you are going to do some advanced poses, such as arm balances or backbends, make sure you practice some basic poses that will prepare your body for these more demanding postures.

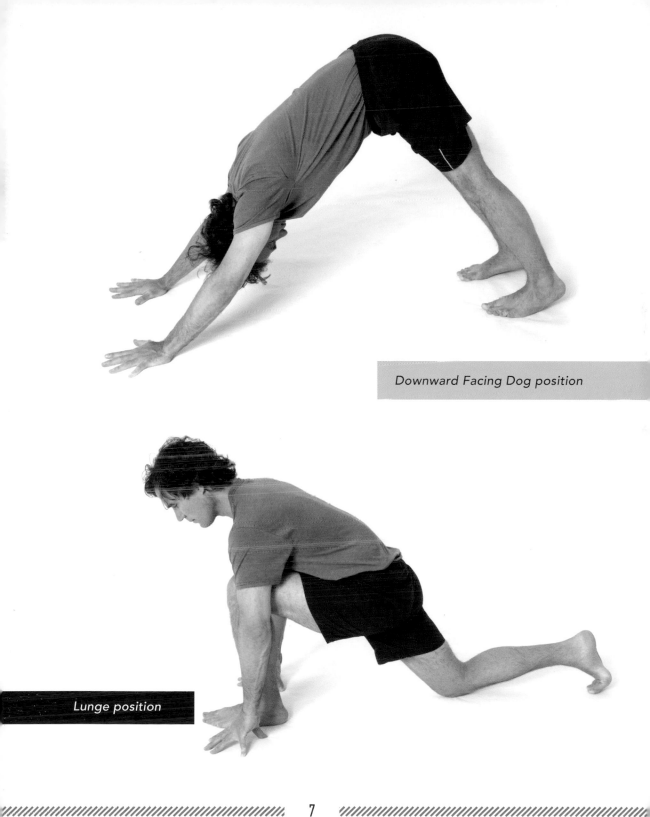

Downward Facing Dog position

Lunge position

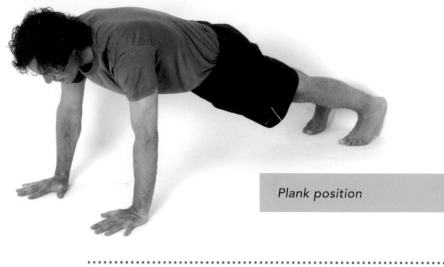

Plank position

Basic Alignment

There are a few basic alignment tips that yogis and yoginis generally adhere to in a wide variety of poses. Because of space limitations, we do not list all of these alignment instructions for each pose. Use these alignment recommendations before you go into a posture, and then maintain the alignment when you are in the pose. Not every alignment technique is applicable for each pose, yet they are for most poses.

HERE ARE SOME OF THEM:

- Lift your lower abs and your lower back up and in toward each other.
- Lift your sternum.
- Relax the top of your shoulders.
- Keep your head in line with your spine.
- Soften your neck and throat.
- Engage your quadriceps.
- Align your shoulders, elbows, and wrists.
- Align your hips, knees, and ankles.
- Breathe evenly. Move on inhalations and exhalations.

Note Mary Dawn's alignment in the photo on the right. Being in alignment makes a big difference in how you feel while doing the posture and afterwards.

It is important to remember that bodies are all a little bit different. Your posture may not look like the models in the book. Thus, it is important to make the suggested adjustments and modify the poses for your body type. Our model, Mary Dawn, has a bit of a sway back. Other people may be knock-kneed or bowlegged. Yoga is not about having the perfect pose. It is about what you experience as you practice the pose. And, yes, it is called yoga *practice*. So you do not have to be perfect.

What Type of Bar Stool Do I Need?

Bar stools come in all shapes and sizes. Here, we use various types of bar stools: different heights, some with backs and some without backs, round seats, and rectangular seats. Different poses work better on shorter stools rather than taller stools. For some postures, a rectangular seat is better. Bar stools with padded seats are great for people who tend to be on the bonier end of the spectrum, particularly if your abdomen is on the stool. Experiment with different bar stools before you commit to a certain type. And if one doesn't work for you, don't use it.

What Do I Wear for Bar Stool Yoga?

Bar stool yoga is a little different from most yoga traditions. As you will see, bar stool yoga can be done in any clothing, from an elegant dress to jeans and a T-shirt to traditional yoga clothes. These days, yoga wear is a norm almost everywhere, particularly for yoginis. And, luckily, there are stretch yoga pants that look just like jeans. So what could be better for a Martini Yogini to wear for a night on the town?

CAUTION

Bar stool yoga is in the tradition of fun yoga. It is meant for a convivial atmosphere with friends: yogis and non-yogis alike. In fact, bar stool yoga encourages everyone to try some yoga, even the simplest poses. Practicing with friends also allows us to spot our friends and for them to spot us, to make sure we are safe.

In some cases, bar stool yoga is almost acrobatic. These poses are only for the most advanced yoga practitioners. Be attentive and alert when performing all yoga poses, and particularly the most advanced postures.

Caution is always advised. Bar stools need to be stable. For many poses, place the stool against a wall or have a friend hold it for you.

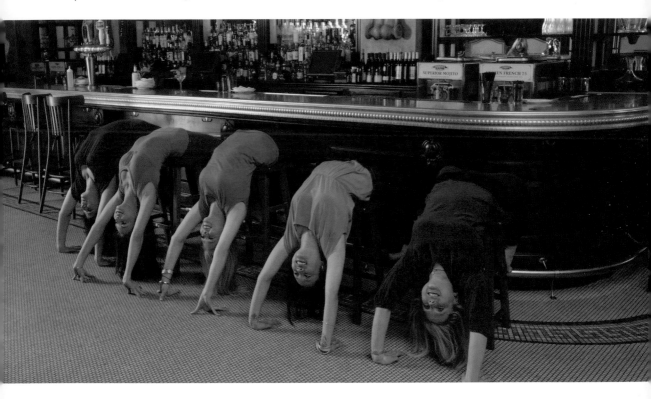

Don't Mix Your Alcohol and Yoga

Bar stool yoga is hip and fantastic. I have had crazy fun dreaming up new names for the poses and photographing them in bars. I want you to try these poses on bar stools with your friends and see how an ordinary evening turns into the most delightful time you have had in a very long time. And most importantly, I sincerely do not want you to hurt yourself by combining your yoga with alcohol. Have fun with the yoga poses on the bar stool, and then have your beer, wine, or cocktails. Always, always, always be safe.

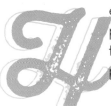ere's a new twist on Girls' Night Out. Try a few of these yoga poses next time you are out on the town. Play "yoga" with your friends, and maybe even impress and entertain some of the other patrons with your equanimity, balance, poise, and sense of fun.

RECIPE FOR A MARTINI YOGINI:

1 PART FUN

1 PART FRIENDLINESS

1 PART SENSE OF ADVENTURE

2 PARTS WISDOM

2 PARTS GRACE

3 PARTS COMPASSION

GARNISH WITH A TWIST OF WHIMSY

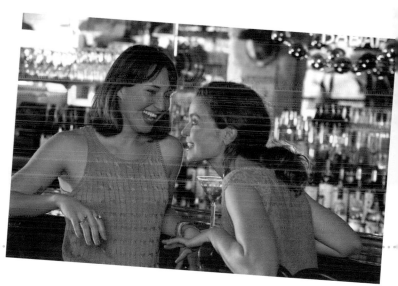

Banana Boat

The traditional Boat Pose is an enjoyable, yet difficult pose that's actually a bit easier on bar stools with backs. You'll need a fair amount of abdominal strength to hold the pose—beer bellies may get in the way. Try this with a friend, preferably someone who is sober, about your height, and who has your level of flexibility.

WHAT YOU DO

1. With a friend, sit on bar stools facing each other.

2. Bend your knees and place the soles of each other's feet together.

3. Hold onto the side of the stool seat, while slowly lifting your legs and straightening your knees.

4. When your legs and torso form approximately a 45-degree angle, take each other's hands and hold on tight.

5. Hold the pose for 15 to 20 seconds at first. Over time, you will be able to hold the position for a minute or longer.

Benefits: This pose builds strength in your lower abs and lower back.

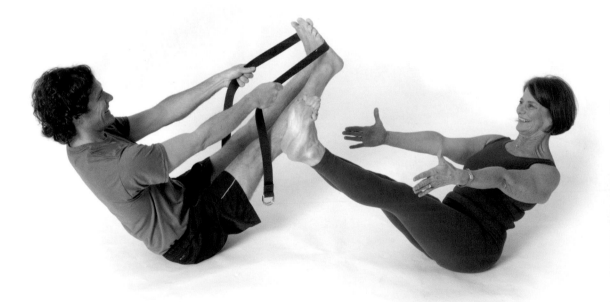

You can practice this pose on the floor by yourself at first. If it's too difficult extending your arms alongside your torso at first, grab someone's necktie and place it around your feet as shown.

Happy Hour Hint

Before you practice this pose, stretch your quadriceps. If your quads are overly tight, this pose will be quite difficult to hold.

Ask Your Bartender For . . .

A Banana Boat, with vanilla ice cream, banana liqueur, crème de cacao, rum, and banana.

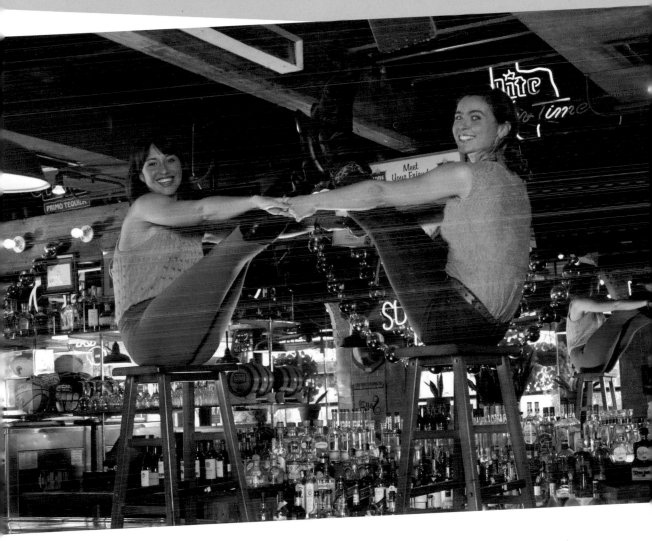

Tipsy Triangle

The classic Triangle pose can be a little tipsy even when you're not. It requires strength, balance, and flexibility all at once, and most of us can only pull off one of the three at any given time.

WHAT YOU DO

1. Stand with your feet 3 ½ to 4 feet apart, depending on your height and flexibility.

2. Turn your right foot out 90 degrees and turn your left foot in about 15 degrees.

3. Align the heel of your forward foot with the arch of your back foot.

4. Extend your arms fully, aligning your hands with your shoulders. Relax the top of your shoulders.

5. Shift your hips to the left. From the right hip crease, laterally move your torso to the right, extending the underside of your torso as much as you extend the top of your torso.

6. Place your right hand on the rung of a bar stool.

7. Place your left hand on your hip. Rotate your torso slightly backward, so your torso, hips, and legs are all in the same plane.

8. Gracefully come out of the pose and switch sides.

Benefits: Triangle strengthens the legs and lower back, tones the abdominal muscles, and increases flexibility in the arms and shoulders.

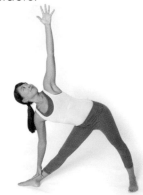

In order to practice this pose at home, follow the same instructions for the bar stool pose. Extend laterally from your hip crease and place your hand on your ankle, the floor, or on a yoga block. Bring your other hand above you, even with your shoulder. Turn your head and look at your hand.

Happy Hour Hint

Use the bar stool rungs to measure your progress with this pose. Reaching the lower rungs means you're gaining flexibility. Just don't overstretch yourself reaching for the floor your first time trying this pose.

Ask Your Bartender For . . .

A Grapefruit Margarita, with tequila, lime, grapefruit, and orange liqueur.

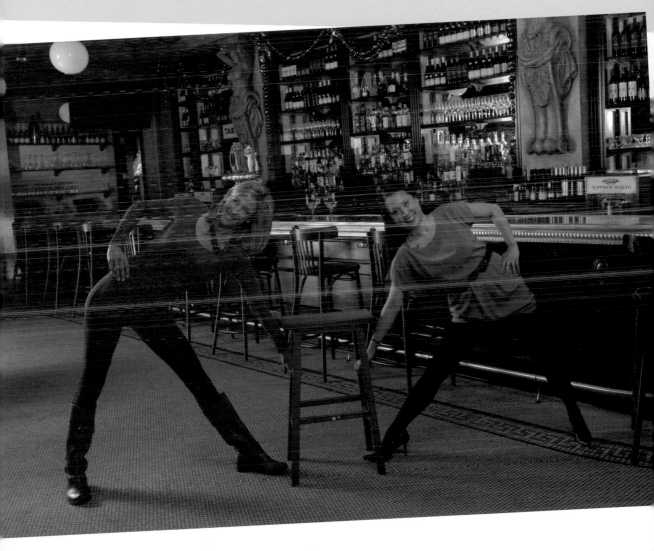

Long Island Iced Tree

Based on the classic Tree pose, you'll use a bar stool to help you balance, which is usually what bar stools are for, anyway. After this pose, enjoy a Long Island Iced Tea, the famous drink created at the Oak Beach Inn on Long Island way back in 1972.

WHAT YOU DO

1. Stand with your feet hip distance apart. Shift your weight to your left leg and foot.

2. Lift your right leg and place the sole of your right foot on your left inner thigh, or as high as possible.

3. Place your right knee on the bar stool.

4. Bring your hands to prayer position at the center of your chest.

5. Hold as long as you like. Gracefully lower your right leg. Repeat the sequence, balancing on your right leg and lifting your left foot.

Benefits: This pose builds strength in the legs and increases the ability to balance.

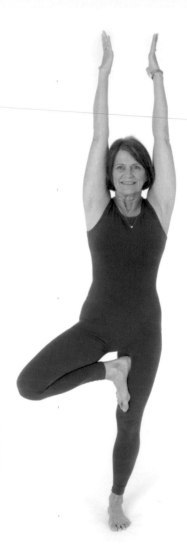

For home practice, the sequence is similar. If you need support, you can place your knee on a wall, rather than on a bar stool seat. If you like, extend your arms overhead, with your arms shoulder-width apart and parallel. To help balance, choose a spot on the wall on which to focus.

Happy Hour Hint

After practicing this technique with a bar stool for support, try it without the stool.

Ask Your Bartender For . . .

A Long Island Iced Tea, of course, which includes triple sec, rum, gin, vodka, tequila, sour mix, and cola. Careful though: it may taste like a refreshing iced tea, but it packs a wallop.

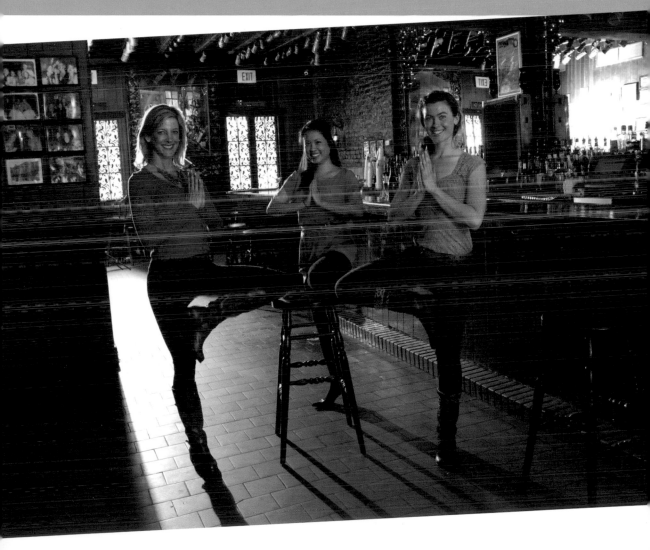

Bar Stool Warrior

Athena, the daughter of Zeus, was born fully-grown from her father's forehead, wearing a full set of armor. You'll feel reborn (and fully dressed for combat) after trying this pose, which is called Warrior III, named after another mythical hero, the Hindu god Virabhadra (who incidentally was also born fully-grown and armored).

WHAT YOU DO

1. Align two bar stools so that the distance between them is the full length of your body with your arms extended.

2. Place your hands on one bar stool.

3. Walk backward until your torso and legs form a right angle.

4. Lift one leg and place it on the stool behind you. Make sure that your front hipbones are even.

5. Hold as long as you like. Gracefully release the pose and switch sides.

Benefits: Builds strength and flexibility in the thighs, hips, torso, and shoulders. Increases ability to balance.

This pose is an extension of Warrior I (page 56). From Warrior I, lean forward and bring your torso over your forward knee. Pause for a moment. Then straighten your forward leg and bring your back leg up, aligning it with your hips. Strongly extend your arms in front of you and your back leg behind you.

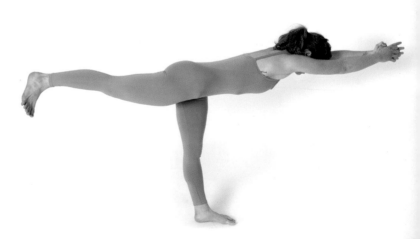

Happy Hour Hint

Lift your lower abs toward your spine in order to prevent your lower back from sinking in the pose. Also, feel free to use only the front bar stool once you think you've got your balance right.

Ask Your Bartender For . . .

An Athenia, which is a Greek cocktail named after Athena. It includes Greek brandy, which is a blend of brandy and wine made from sun-dried grapes; champagne; orange liqueur; and orange juice. Drink with caution, otherwise you'll wake up feeling like Zeus after giving birth to Athena.

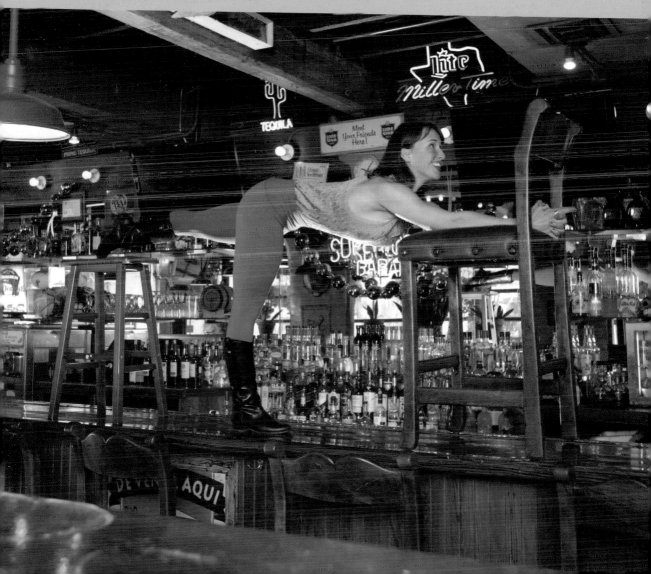

Weekend Warrior

Weekends can be jammed packed with fun, exercise, errands, family commitments, and more. You have got to pace yourself so you won't feel exhausted by Monday morning. Before hitting the pub for that well-earned drink or two, practice some Warrior poses with your yogini friends.

WHAT YOU DO

1. Stand facing forward with a bar stool on your right side. Widen your feet so they are 4 feet apart.

2. Turn your right foot out 90 degrees and turn your left foot inward approximately 15 degrees. Align the heel of your forward foot with the arch of your back foot.

3. Place your right foot on the lowest rung of the bar stool. Bend your right knee into a right angle.

4. Hold as long as you want. Gracefully release and switch sides, repeating with your left foot on the bar stool rung.

Benefits: Builds strength and flexibility in the legs, lower back, and lower abdomen.

This pose is almost identical to the Bar Stool version, except that both feet are on the floor.

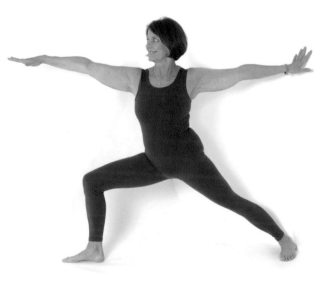

Happy Hour Hint

Placing the ball of your forward foot on a folded mat during this pose can help heal knee pain. You can also place your forward foot on a yoga block, the rung of a bar stool, or a chair seat, all which allow more ease of movement in your hip joint.

Ask Your Bartender For . . .

A Warrior, which is a strong drink consisting of vermouth, brandy, anise-flavored liqueur, and orange liqueur.

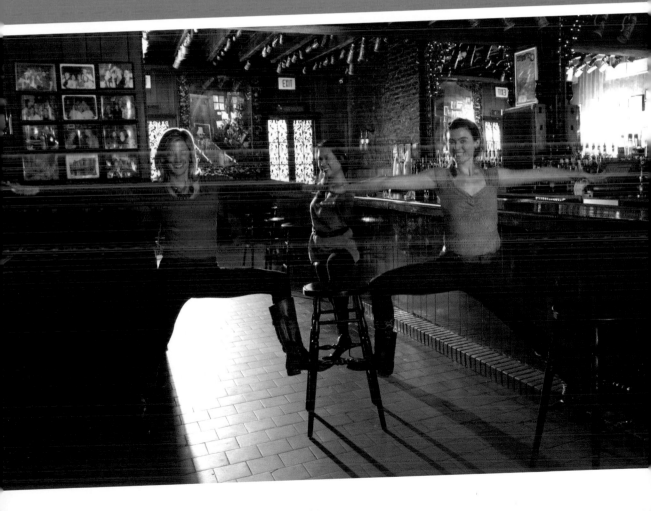

Cyclone

Martini Yoginis might just create a Cyclone, which is a much more interesting name for Camel pose. Why? Because Martini Yoginis blow in, practice a few poses, and blow out faster than a hurricane.

WHAT YOU DO

1. Grab a buddy as this pose is much more fun with a friend.

2. Kneel in front of a low bar stool without a backrest, with your knees and feet together and the top of your feet on the floor. You may have to visit several bars before finding just the right bar stool for this pose.

3. Bring the stool seat to your back.

4. Place your hands on your hips. Tighten your glutes. Lean backward, placing your back on the stool seat, and bring your head down and back.

5. Bring your hands behind your head, catching your friend's hands.

6. Hold for 30 to 60 seconds, breathing evenly.

7. To release, slowly come up, leading with your chest and bringing your head up last. Rest for a moment, so you do not become dizzy.

Benefits: The back muscles are stretched and strengthened. Plus, backbends very often help relieve respiratory issues.

The traditional pose is very similar to the bar stool pose, except when you curve your spine backward and drop your head, place your hands on your feet or ankles. While you are in the pose, continually lift your chest toward the ceiling.

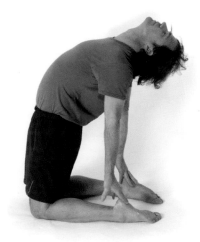

Happy Hour Hint

Practicing this pose over a low bar stool is very beneficial for those who are new to yoga or who have injuries. The bar stool supports you, giving you many of the benefits of the pose without the undue strain a beginner might experience.

Ask Your Bartender For . . .

There are lots of recipes for Cyclone cocktails, but legend has it that the first cyclone drinks were created at Pat O'Brien's in the French Quarter in New Orleans, not long after they created The Hurricane. One such fruity recipe calls for amaretto, grenadine syrup, Jack Daniel's, and orange juice.

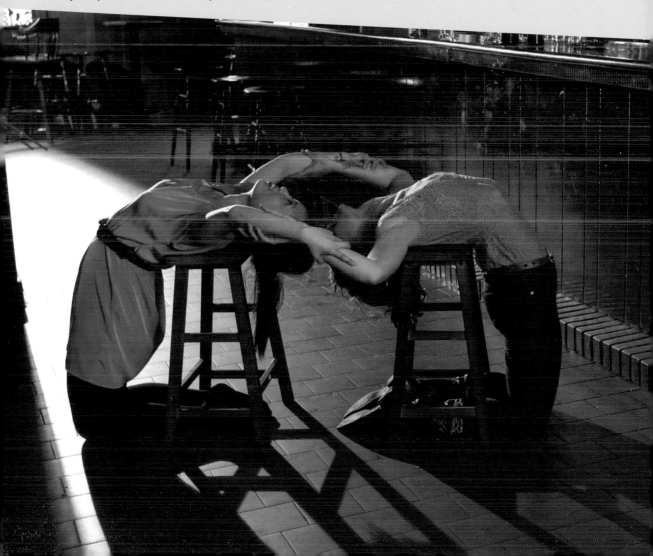

Blue Dolphin Plank

Dolphin Plank with your girlfriends at the bar: It's a great pose for chatting. Meanwhile, you can drink all the Blue Dolphins you want—it's a shot glass full of water, meant as a joke.

WHAT YOU DO

1. Interlock your fingers and allow about 4 inches of space between your palms.

2. Place the sides of your hands and the sides of your forearms on the seat of the bar stool. Align your shoulders and your elbows.

3. Walk your feet back until your body is in a straight line.

4. Meanwhile, lift your shoulders and bring your tummy and your lower back in toward each other.

5. Engage all of your leg muscles and press your heels toward the wall behind you. Look at your friends or at the bar stool.

6. To release, walk your feet toward the bar stool.

Benefits: Builds strength in the arms, shoulders, and core.

For at-home practice, kneel on a yoga mat. The basic instructions are the same as the bar stool pose, except that your body will be parallel with the floor.

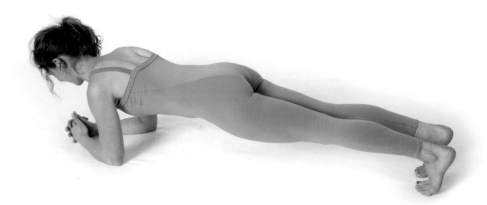

Happy Hour Hint

If you're a beginner, practice this pose first with your feet against a wall or the bar. Press your heels firmly into the wall or bar as you do the pose. This helps stabilize your core.

Ask Your Bartender For . . .

A zingy Blue Dolphin Martini, with vodka, blue curacao liqueur, and peach schnapps.

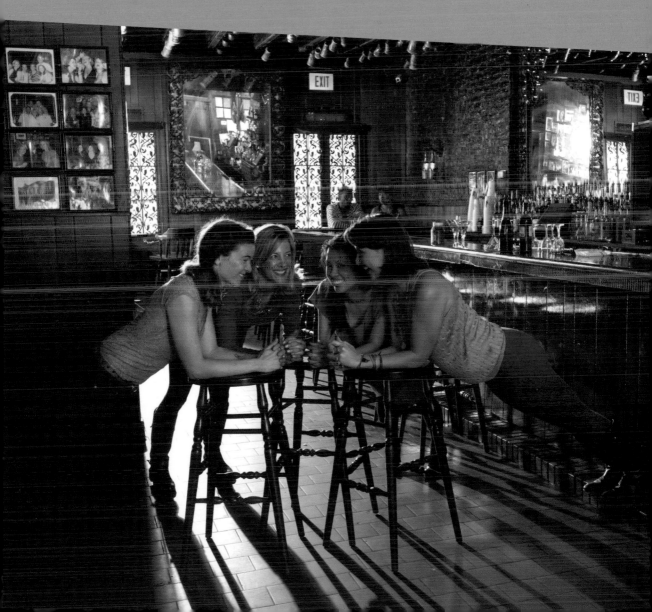

Link-Up

At the end of the night, everyone is linking up, finalizing the evening by combining a very special cocktail with a friendly, feel-good pose.

WHAT YOU DO

1. Sit on a bar stool with your legs extended in front of you and your feet together on another bar stool seat.

2. Lift your arms overhead.

3. Bend forward from your hip crease.

4. Extend from the base of your spine as evenly as possible and extend your sternum toward your feet.

5. Hold your friends' hands and help each other extend just a little bit more. Just don't pull each other off your stools.

Benefits: Stretches the hamstrings and the back. Allows the mind to quiet (when not done in a bar).

The directions are the same for home linking up except you are on the floor. Most beginners cannot reach their toes, so place a yoga strap around your feet and hold the strap at a length that is right for your level of flexibility.

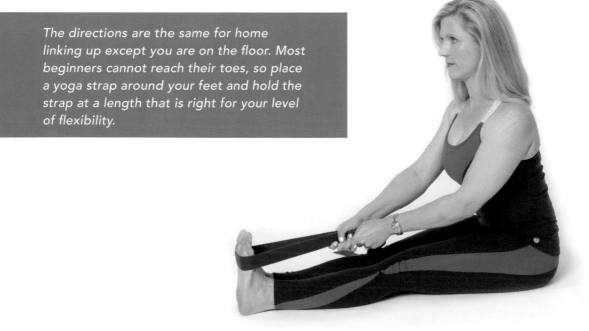

Happy Hour Hint

When practicing this pose, allow your torso to gradually release toward your feet, rather than forcing further extension.

Ask Your Bartender For . . .

A Link Up, which is a cocktail created by the famous bartender, Joe Gilmore, at the American Bar in London in 1975. This mixture of American whiskey and Russian vodka honored the first joint space mission between the United States and the Union of Soviet Socialist Republics. Of course, the drink is served over ice.

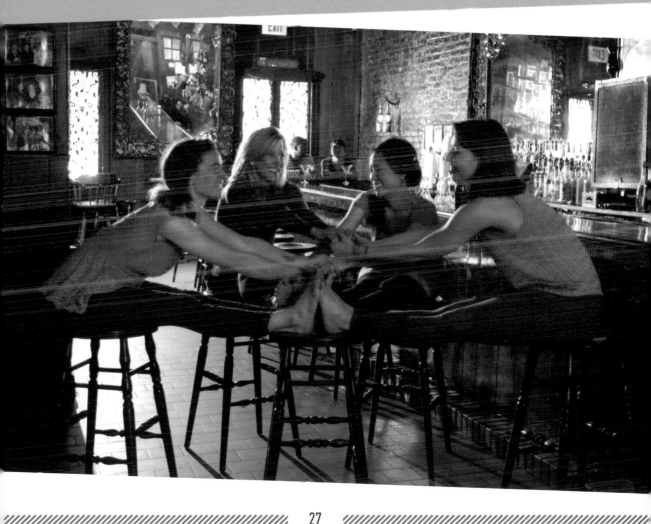

CHAPTER 2
TOO MANY TEQUILA SUN(RISE) SALUTATIONS

Too many Tequila Sunrises last night resulting in too much coffee the next morning and a need for some Sun Salutations to get the blood flowing again? Wake up your buddies from the night before, tell them to put on some comfortable clothing, and meet you at the coffee bar for some seriously fun Sun Salutes.

RECIPE FOR A TEQUILA SUN(RISE) SALUTATION:

1 PART GRANITE RESOLVE

1 PART COMPASSION FOR SELF

1 PART SILLINESS

2 PARTS LOVE

COFFEE, LOTS OF GREAT COFFEE

ICE AND ASPIRIN (OPTIONAL)

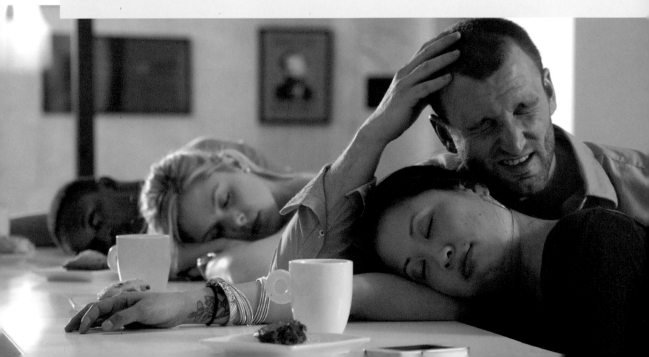

Salty Dog

Maybe it really was the tequila last night, or perhaps there's something funky in your morning muffin. Either way, Downward Facing Dog has never been this much fun. When practicing with friends, delight in playing around with the pose. If in class, or practicing at home, try the more traditional method and spice it up with some hints that help with alignment, lightness, and joy.

WHAT YOU DO

1. It is best to have stools that are fixed to the floor, so the stools don't slide. Ideally, there should be three stools. (See photo on next page.)

2. Kneel on all fours with your hands on one stool, knees on the middle stool, and feet on the third.

3. Arch your lower back. Lift your hips and straighten your legs. Your torso and your legs will form a 45- to 50-degree angle. Drop your head.

4. Stretch as fully as you can, extending your spine.

5. Hold for 30 to 60 seconds. Release carefully.

6. For fun, a friend can do a modified Dog pose, using your back and another stool (like in the photo on the next page). Just be careful.

Benefits: Strengthens and stretches the arms, legs, shoulders, and spine.

The traditional pose is performed basically the same way. To keep the weight in the back of your body, press your thighs toward the wall behind you and actively push your heels into the floor.

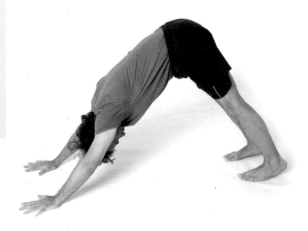

Happy Hour Hint

Bringing most of your weight to your legs will make the pose effortless on your arms and shoulders. The following variations will accomplish that desired effect when doing the traditional pose: a) Place a folded yoga mat under your heels and press your heels into the mat; b) Place your heels on a wall and press them into the wall; c) Place your hands on yoga blocks, which will help you get your heels to the floor more easily.

Ask Your Bartender For . . .

A Salty Dog, which includes grapefruit juice, gin, and salt.

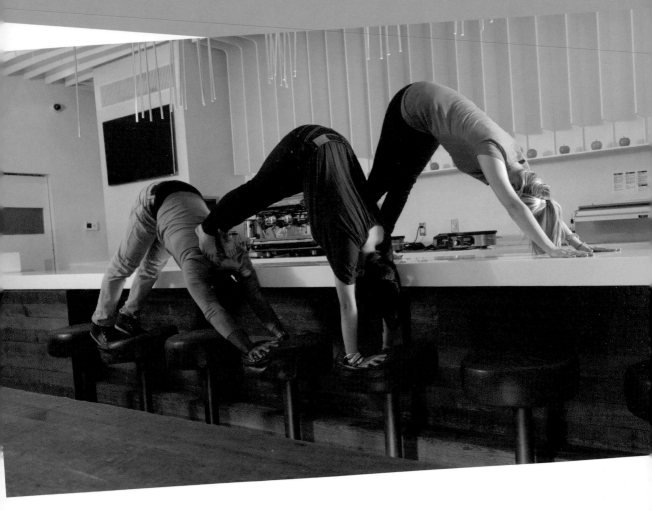

Leap-Frog Lunge

Before you leap, lunge, or crawl for that extra cup of coffee and aspirin, try this pose, which will do wonders for your energy. Lunge is normally done as part of the Sun Salutations from Downward Dog. The main instructions below are for the Revolved Lunge; however, you can start off with a regular Lunge. (Instructions are included with the traditional pose steps below.)

WHAT YOU DO

1. Once again, this pose is best done with stools that are fixed to the floor. (See photo on next page.)

2. From Downward Dog (see page 7), step your right foot forward between your hands, aligning your right knee over your ankle.

3. Lower your left knee to the stool behind you and slide the knee back until you feel a comfortable stretch in your left front thigh.

4. Gently revolve your torso toward your forward leg.

5. Place your hands in prayer position at your heart.

6. Hold the pose as long as you like. To release, come back into Downward Facing Dog. Then repeat with your left leg forward.

Benefits: Stretches the thighs, builds strength in the back muscles, and improves overall energy.

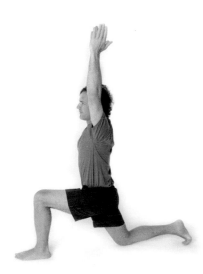

To practice the traditional pose at home, start in Downward Dog, and then follow the directions for the bar stool pose. But instead of revolving, bring your arms overhead, shoulder-width apart. For the Revolved Lunge, twist from the very bottom of your spine. Your knee can be up or on the floor in either variation of Lunge pose.

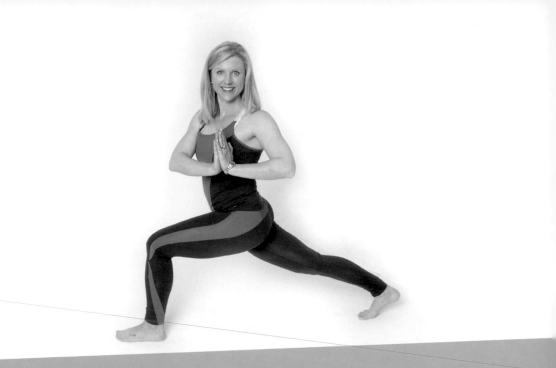

In some cases, such as in the image below, the stools won't be the right distance for your height. Just do the best you can; however, if you feel uncomfortable, move to the floor and do the traditional pose. Or, with permission, use the coffee bar.

Ask Your Bartender For . . .

A Leap Frog, which is a traditional British cocktail, made of gin, ginger ale, and lemon juice. If the yoga and coffee aren't making you feel better, this should do the trick.

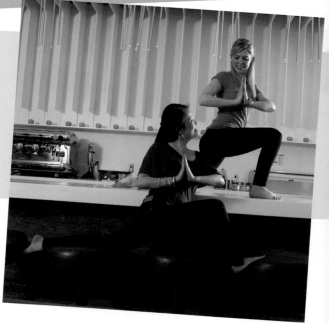

Painkiller Plank

If anything will cure overindulgence, it has got to be this version of Plank pose. Or maybe you will need a Painkiller cocktail after this pose … not really sure.

WHAT YOU DO

1. In this version of Plank pose, align a table and a bar stool—your body's width apart. (See photo on page 35.)

2. Start by placing your hands on the bar stool and feet on the floor.

3. Walk your feet up to the tabletop. You will be on your toes, with your heels stretching toward the wall behind you.

4. Adjust yourself so your shoulders are aligned over your wrists.

5. Lift your arms and shoulders maximally. Bring your lower back and lower abs in toward each other. Firm your legs. Hold as long as you like.

6. If a friend wants to do Plank pose on your back, have him or her tread very carefully.

Benefits: Builds strength in the arms, shoulders, legs, and core.

For the traditional Plank pose, follow the directions above, but place your feet against a wall, and don't invite anyone onto your back.

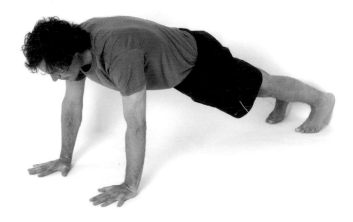

For Side Forearm Plank, start with Forearm Plank pose with both forearms on the floor.

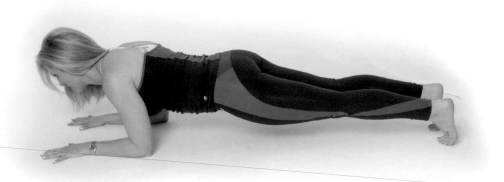

Shift your weight to your left arm and rotate your torso to the right. Release by coming back into full Forearm Plank. Repeat on the other side. Keep your legs firm and strongly press your heels toward the wall behind you, as you place the side of the top foot on the side of the bottom foot. Keep your legs and torso firm.

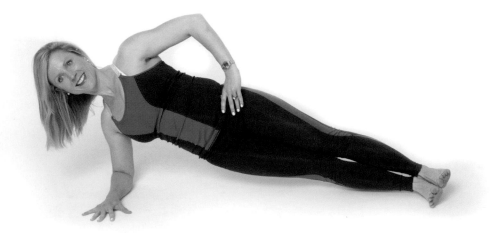

Happy Hour Hint

Both versions of Plank can be done more easily and accurately with your feet firmly pressing into a wall.

Ask Your Bartender For . . .

The Painkiller cocktail, which originated at the Soggy Dollar Bar located on an isolated beach on the island of Jost Van Dyke in the British Virgin Islands. There's no dock, so the usual way to get there is to swim. Of course, your dollars get wet—hence the name. The cocktail, with the refreshing tastes of coconut cream, pineapple juice, and dark rum, may be what caused the need for these energizing Plank poses. Life can be a vicious cycle.

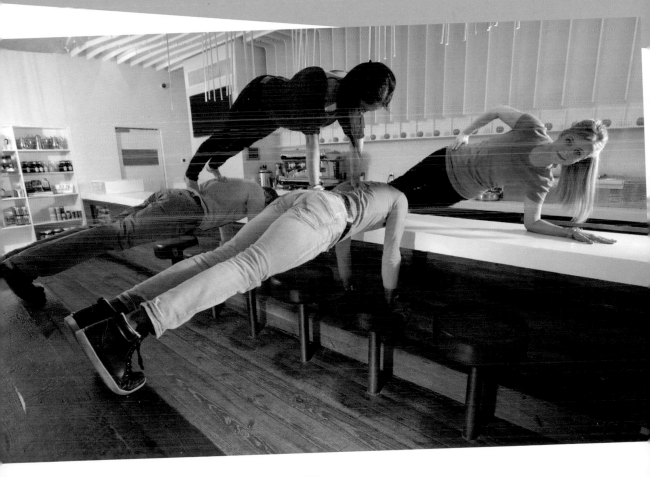

Plank on the Rocks

The image on the opposite page shows two different poses. While Randy and Jimmy are doing an intense, two-legged Plank pose, Van and Kristen are doing their goddess impersonations in Rock pose. Rock pose is a standard in Kundalini Yoga. The pose gets its name from the assertion that the pose is so good for digestion that if you practice it regularly, you will be able to eat and easily digest rocks … or tequila on the rocks.

WHAT YOU DO

FOR THE ROCK POSE

1. Kneel with the tops of your feet on the floor. Make sure that your knees, ankles, and feet are touching.

2. Sit back on your heels. Hold the pose as long as you like.

FOR THE TWO-LEGGED PLANK POSE

1. From Downward Dog, come into Plank pose (see page 8) by shifting your torso forward so your shoulders are directly over your wrists.

2. Keep your lower abs and your lower back firm and moving toward each other and your thighs firm.

3. Keep your entire body—hips, spine, and neck—in one line.

4. Then, lift one arm and the opposite leg, extending them as much as possible.

5. Hold for 20 to 30 seconds. Release, reestablish Plank pose and lift the other arm and leg.

Benefits: Rock pose aids in digestion and gives a sense of wellbeing and calmness, while the Two-legged Plank pose builds strength in the arms, shoulders, legs, and core.

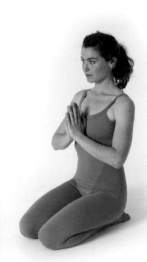

Rock pose is practiced the same way whether at a coffee bar or at home.

Happy Hour Hint

If the Rock pose is difficult on your knees, place a folded blanket between your calves and thighs. If they still hurt, place a folded blanket on your heels. If your ankles hurt, try a rolled face towel underneath each anklebone. Experiment with the width of the rolled towel, making sure you get the optimal comfort for your ankles.

Ask Your Bartender For . . .

A Walk the Plank, which consists of spiced rum, coconut rum, blue curacao liqueur, and pineapple juice.

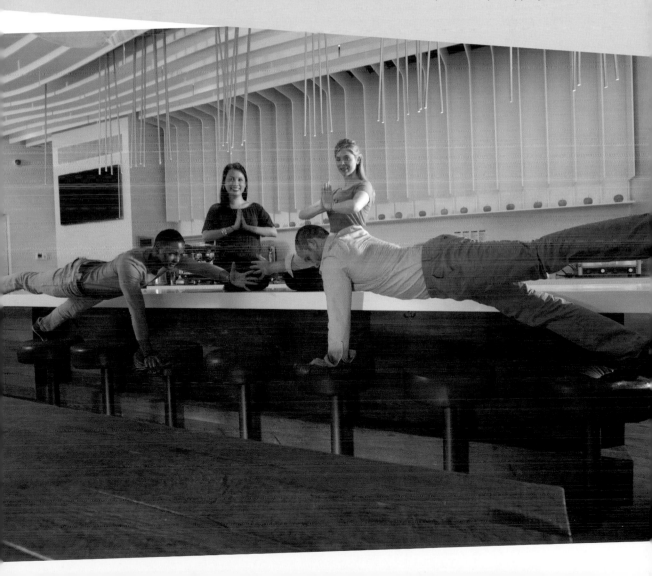

Hell, Yeah!

You've stretched and practiced the poses in this chapter, and yes, by golly, you've got your swagger back. What? Not quite there yet? No worries. Try a few backbends. Backbends expand the chest and lungs, allowing more oxygen intake. This alone increases your energy. Plus, the pose strengthens your arms, shoulders, legs, spine, and back muscles. No wonder backbends feel so great!

WHAT YOU DO

1. Lie on the bar on your back. Bend your knees and place your feet, hip-width apart, as close to your hips as possible.

2. Place your palms, shoulder-width apart, on either side of your head. Your fingers will face your shoulders. Lift your back off the bar and place the crown of your head on the bar.

3. Roll your thighs inward and press the back of your thighs toward the front of your thighs.

4. Straighten your arms and legs, arch your back, and propel your torso toward the ceiling.

5. Lift your heels and stretch your back and abdomen toward the ceiling. Then carefully place your heels on the bar.

6. Firm your hips and push them and your entire back toward the ceiling. Continually curve your spine inward, toward your chest and toward the ceiling.

7. Hold for as long as you like. Slowly come down, first placing the crown of your head on the bar. Then release completely and rest on the bar, without pulling your knees to your chest or doing any type of forward bend. Repeat as many times as you like. When completely finished with your backbends, perform some forward bends.

Benefits: Strengthens and increases flexibility in the back, legs, shoulders, and arms. Enhances suppleness in the spine.

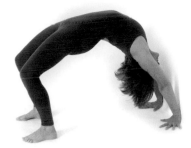

For at-home practice, continually lift the back of your body toward the front of your body and the front of your body toward the ceiling.

Happy Hour Hint

Once you've practiced this pose a bit, focus on rolling the outside edge of your armpits and your deltoid muscles toward each other and sliding your shoulder blades toward your hips. Then try rolling your thighs inward, toward each other, as you lift them toward the ceiling. With these adjustments, your pose will feel almost effortless. Breathe smoothly and evenly throughout the pose.

Ask Your Bartender For . . .

The Hell, Yeah! cocktail, which is popular in Australia, consists of a juniper-flavored gin, another gin that is steeped with herbs, raspberry juice, fresh lime, and ginger beer.

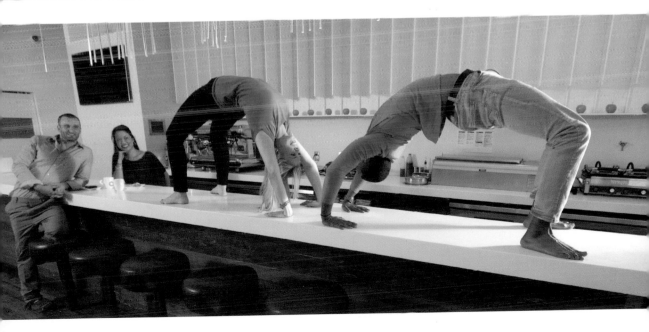

CHAPTER 3
SHAKEN, NOT STIRRED

It's inevitable. You invite a friend over and she wants to show you the cool things she has learned in yoga class. Before you know it, everyone is in on the act—trying yoga poses without ever having gone to a class, surprising themselves, and doing things they never imagined. And having a blast "playing yoga" on a bar stool. When James Bond says, "Shaken, not stirred," he is referring to his martini. But in yoga, we are shaking things up in our bodies, minds, and spirits—and feeling fantastic.

RECIPE FOR SHAKING THINGS UP:

3 PARTS FRIENDS
1 PART OPENNESS
2 PARTS SENSE OF ADVENTURE
GARNISH WITH LAUGHTER

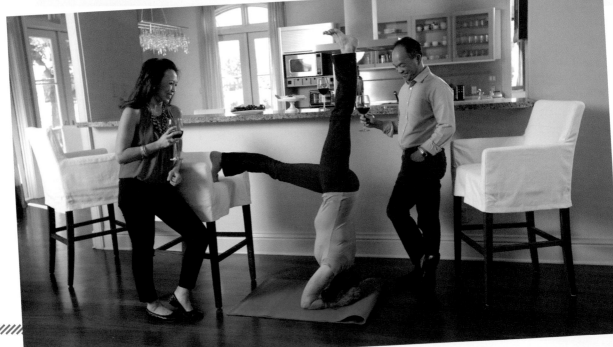

B&B

It's one thing to bond with a friend, but imagine staring at them while practicing Bound Baddha Konasana, or Bound Angle pose. This could certainly shake things up and your friendship could reach new depths. Or it could have the two of you reaching for drinks sooner rather than later. This pose should be done with your back as straight as possible. (That's why in the image on the next page, Nancy is helping Diem lift his chest, which in turn helps lift the upper back.) This version of the pose is particularly helpful if you have stiffness in your legs, hips, and lower back.

WHAT YOU DO

1. With a friend, sit on bar stools with another bar stool between you. (See photo on next page.)

2. Place the soles of your feet together or place your feet around your friend's feet.

3. Press the soles of your feet together, and continue that movement throughout the pose.

4. Continually lift your lower back, lower abdomen, and sternum.

5. Stay in the pose for up to five minutes.

Benefits: This pose is great for stretching your inner thighs, relieving knee pain, and giving energy when you are tired.

To do the traditional pose, sit on the floor with the soles of your feet together, and firmly press them together. If you have trouble keeping your spine and chest lifted, place your hands behind your back and press your hands or fingers into the floor.

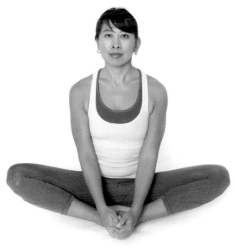

If your hips and inner thighs are tight, try the pose sitting on a bar stool with your feet on a stool in front of you. Otherwise, try the traditional pose seated on a folded blanket or two.

Ask Your Bartender For . . .

A B&B, in which you float brandy on top of Benedictine herbal liqueur.

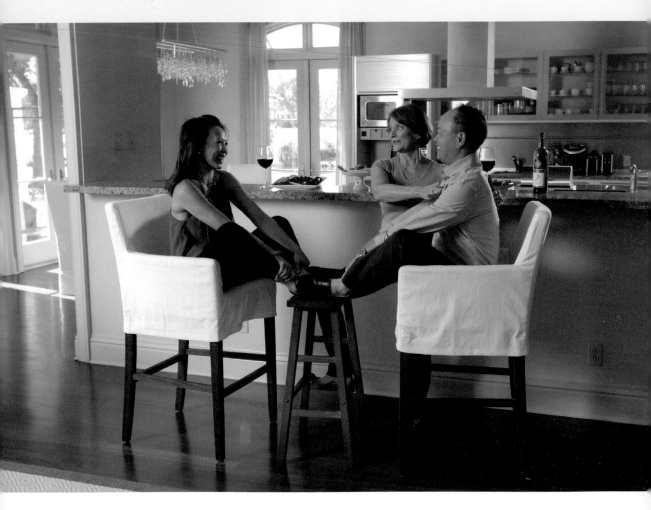

Bahama Mama

Bahama Mamas naturally want to nurture their babies, and do so with Rock the Baby pose. Okay, so maybe those toes make an ugly baby face, but your hips and lower back will surely feel good when you finish rockin'. (And remember, don't drink a Bahama Mama while rocking a real baby!)

WHAT YOU DO

1. Sit on a bar stool, and bring your right foot in toward you.

2. Place your foot either in your left hand or in the crook of your left elbow, depending on your level of flexibility.

3. Continually lift your spine while keeping your shoulders relaxed.

4. Bring your calf as high as your heart, or as close to it as possible. Move your leg from side to side, as though you are rocking a baby.

5. Rock for about one minute.

6. Release and switch sides, repeating all of the instructions above.

Benefits: This pose increases flexibility in the hips and lower back. Feels great!

When performing this posture on the floor, keep one leg firmly extended. It is more difficult to keep your spine straight when you are on the floor, so continually lift your spine as you rock that baby.

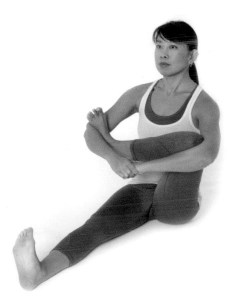

Happy Hour Hint

If you cannot place your foot in the crook of your elbow, place your foot in your hand and practice this way until you gain the flexibility to bring your leg in closer.

Ask Your Bartender For . . .

A Bahama Mama, with dark rum, 151-proof rum, coffee liqueur, coconut liqueur, lemon juice, and pineapple juice.

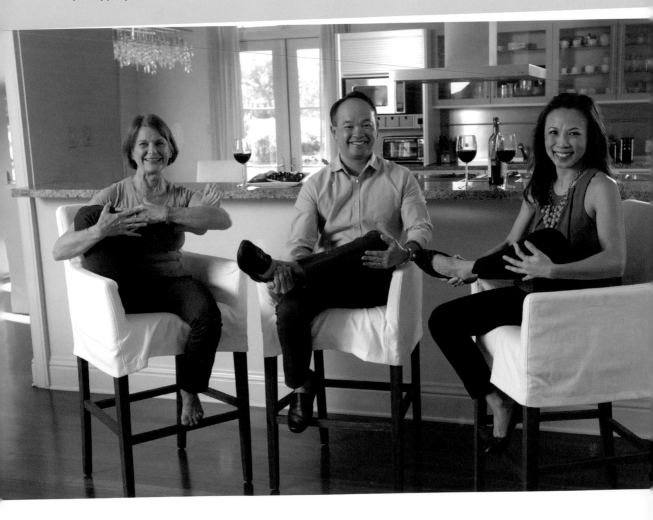

Moscow Mule

Normally called Right Angle pose, we renamed this pose after the famous drink, created by a ginger beer marketer and his buddies. This pose is great for your flexibility, even if it does look like the position you could be in if you drink too many Moscow Mules.

WHAT YOU DO

1. Place your hands on a bar stool seat. (See photo on next page.)

2. Walk back until your torso and legs form a right angle. Your legs should be hip-distance apart and your hands aligned with your shoulders.

3. One friend can hold your lower abs and lower back, to remind you to bring the two toward each other. The other friend can help you hold steady (or steady the bar stool).

4. Extend your spine as much as you can, and press your thighs toward the wall behind you.

5. Keep your head in line with your spine and hold as long as you like.

6. Release by walking in toward the chair.

Benefits: Increases flexibility in your spine, back muscles, arms, shoulders, and legs.

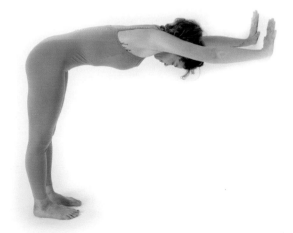

For home practice, place your hands on a wall, waist high. Then follow the directions for the bar stool pose. Press your hands into the wall, as though you are trying to knock the wall over. This will increase the stretch of your back muscles and spine.

Happy Hour Hint

Try this pose with friends helping you.

Ask Your Bartender For . . .

A Moscow Mule, which consists of either ginger beer or ginger ale, vodka, and a lemon wedge.

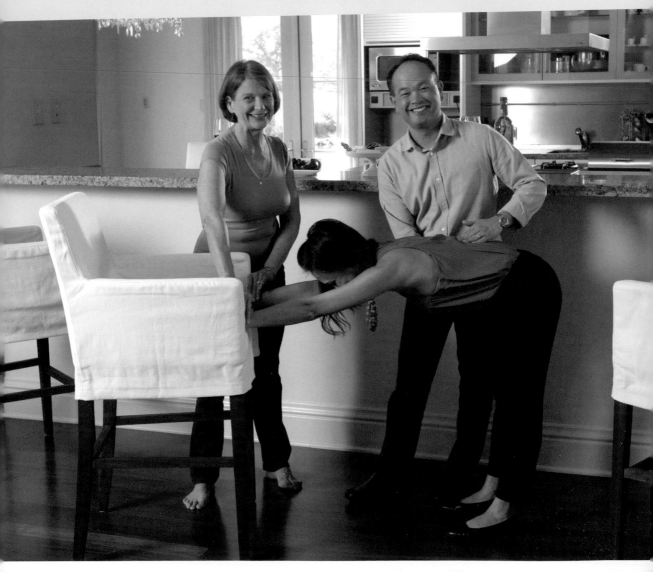

Moonwalk

Imagine how easy Right Angle Handstand pose is in zero gravity. In honor of the first moon landing in 1969, this "giant leap for mankind," we have renamed this pose after the historic event (as well as the celebratory cocktail—see page 48). Until we can all enjoy zero gravity, take your time with this pose, as gravity won't be your friend at first.

WHAT YOU DO

1. Place the bar stool against a wall or have a friend steady it.

2. Sit with your back at the bar stool and your feet stretched forward.

3. Mark where your ankles are. Your hands will be placed approximately there. You may have to experiment a couple of times to get the right spot. The goal is that your torso and your legs form a right angle.

4. Facing away from the bar stool, place your hands, shoulder-width apart, where your ankles were. The heel of your hands will be facing the wall. Spread your fingers wide and firmly and evenly press your hands into the floor.

5. Walk your feet up the bar stool and place your toes and balls of your feet on the seat. Extend your heels toward the back of the bar stool.

6. Lift every arm muscle from the wrists to the shoulders.

7. Lengthen your spine and stretch your torso evenly. Allow your head to hang, softening your neck muscles.

8. Hold as long as you can. To release, walk your feet down the bar stool. Lean forward for a minute or two, to prevent dizziness.

Benefits: This pose strengthens your arms, legs, and upper body and stretches your shoulders.

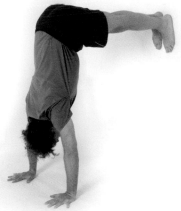

For home practice, sit against a wall with your legs extended. Mark where your ankles are and place your hands there, shoulder-distance apart. Walk your feet up the wall until your legs and torso form a right angle. Press your feet firmly into the wall and lift every arm muscle, from the wrists to the shoulders.

Happy Hour Hint

This pose is a beginner handstand pose and is more difficult than it appears. It requires less flexibility and more strength than a traditional handstand. Practice this pose for a few weeks or months before attempting a full handstand.

Ask Your Bartender For . . .

A Moonwalk, which was created by legendary bartender, Joe Gilmore, at the American Bar at the Savoy Hotel in London, to commemorate the first moon landing in July 1969. The drink is a combination of grapefruit, orange liqueur, and a hint of rosewater, topped with champagne, and it was the first thing Neil Armstrong and Buzz Aldrin drank upon returning to Earth.

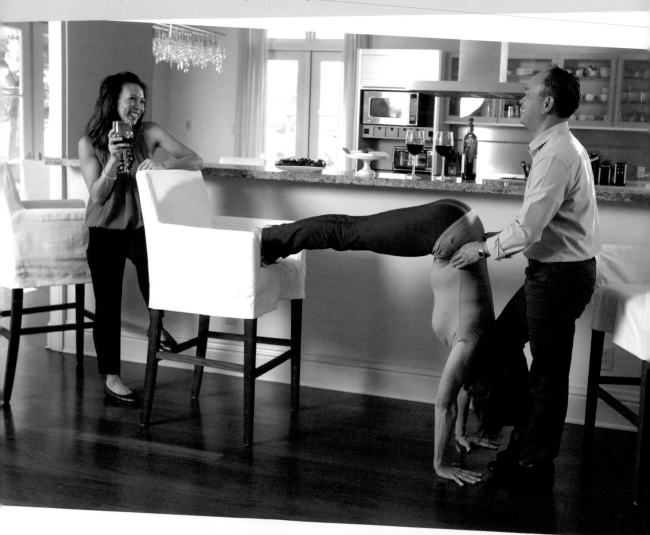

Harvey Headbanger

Be sure not to bang your head in this pose! This variation of Right Angle Head-stand is a safe way to start a headstand practice.

WHAT YOU DO

1. If you are inexperienced in this pose, place your bar stool against a wall and have a friend help you.

2. Sit with your back at the edge of the bar stool and mark where your ankles are. Your head will be placed approximately there. You may have to experiment a couple of times to get the right spot.

3. Kneel and place the sides of your forearms on the floor. Interlock your fingers so they form a "basket," and place the back of your head in the basket and the crown of your head on the floor.

4. Lift your shoulders as much as you can and still keep your head on the floor.

5. Walk your feet up the bar stool until your toes are on the seat. Actively press your heels toward the wall behind you.

6. Start by holding about 30 seconds and working up to holding for 5 minutes at a time.

7. To release, come down slowly and rest with your head down for a minute or two.

Benefits: Headstand has so many benefits that it is considered the king of all the poses. It tones and strengthens the body, improves circulation (particularly to the brain), and increases the function of the glandular system.

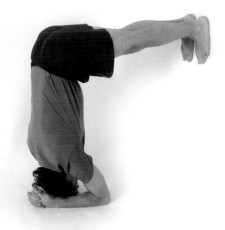

When using the wall instead of the bar stool, press your feet firmly into the wall.

Do not practice this pose if you have high or low blood pressure or if you have spinal issues, particularly in your neck. Initially practice this pose with the help of a very qualified yoga instructor. And, definitely, do not drink alcohol and do this pose!

Ask Your Bartender For . . .

A Harvey Wallbanger, which consists of vodka, Italian herbal liqueur, and orange juice.

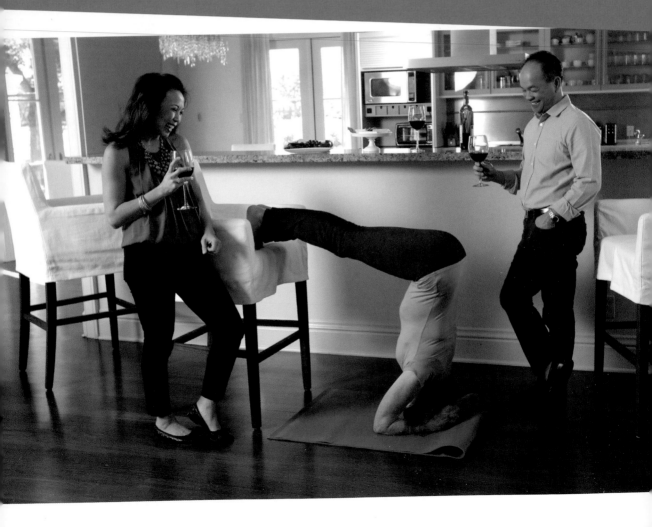

Planter's Punch Padmasana

If you are new to Padmasana, Lotus pose, you should practice this on the floor before attempting on a bar stool. If your legs and/or hips are on the stiff side, practice some other hip opening poses prior to attempting Padmasana. As you advance in the pose, you can sit this way almost anywhere, making all your friends jealous.

WHAT YOU DO

1. Sit tall, with your lower back and lower abdomen lifted.

2. Bend your right leg and hold your foot with your hands.

3. Place your foot at the very top of the left thigh, in the hip crease.

4. Bend your left leg and place the left foot at the very top of your right thigh, near your hip crease.

5. Hold for as long as you like and switch legs.

Benefits: This pose helps to increase flexibility in the knees, ankles, and hips. It also increases circulation in the lower back and abdomen. Lotus is a primary pose used for meditation because it helps calm the mind and the nervous system.

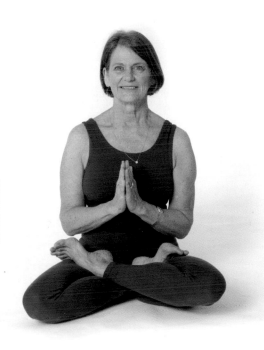

The directions for doing this pose on the mat are identical to the bar stool pose.

Happy Hour Hint

If your knees hurt, place a small, rolled facecloth behind your knees. If your knees continue to hurt, perhaps you need to practice other poses that increase flexibility in the hips and knees. Another trick to getting into the pose more easily is to sit on the edge of two or three folded blankets.

Ask Your Bartender For . . .

Planter's Punch, which is made of dark rum, lemon juice, grenadine syrup, and a dash of bitters. The recipe first appeared in print in a 1908 edition of the *New York Times.* Like many other drinks, it has a disputed origin: one claim refers to the Planters Inn in Charleston, South Carolina, another to the Planter's Hotel in St. Louis, Missouri, and yet another tells of a Jamaican planter's wife who concocted it to cool down the workers.

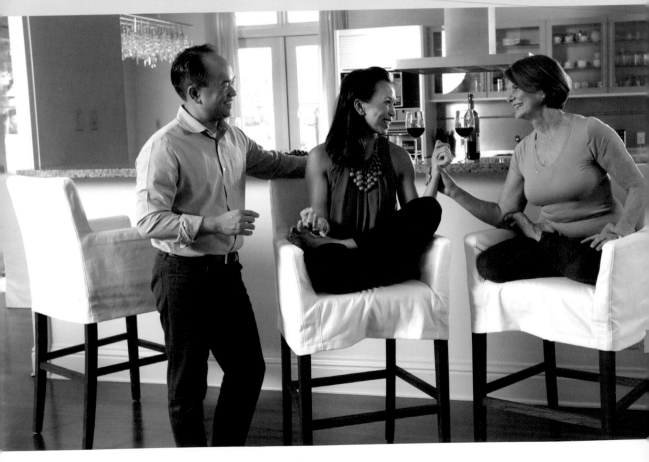

Singapore Swing

The Raffles Hotel in Singapore claims to have invented the Singapore Sling cocktail in 1915. We renamed Tolasana pose to Singapore Swing just now— to celebrate lifting your spirits as well as your body. The pose is traditionally performed sitting on the floor, but using a bar stool that has arms higher than your hips makes it easier to lift yourself.

WHAT YOU DO

1. Sit in Padmasana (Lotus) and place your hands on the arms of the bar stool. (See photo on next page.) On an exhalation, straighten your arms and lift your hips. If you feel strong in the pose, swing back and forth.

2. Release by bending your arms. Release your legs and recross them with the other leg on top. Straighten your arms and lift yourself again.

Benefits: In addition to the benefits of Padmasana, this pose strengthens the hands, arms, shoulders, and abdominal muscles.

The directions for the traditional pose are the same as the bar stool pose, except your hands will be on the floor, which will make it a little more difficult to lift yourself. If you need some help (or if you have short arms), place some yoga blocks under your hands.

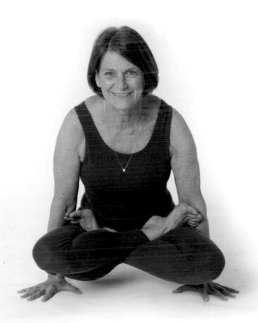

Happy Hour Hint

To enjoy this pose if you cannot perform full Lotus, simply cross your ankles, as Trinh and Diem do in the image below, and then lift yourself.

Ask Your Bartender For . . .

A Singapore Sling, which includes gin, cherry brandy, pineapple juice, lime juice, orange liqueur, Benedictine herbal liqueur, grenadine, and bitters.

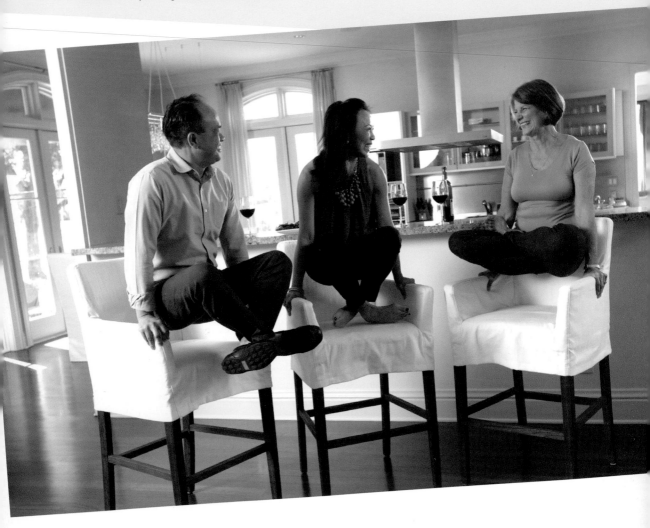

CHAPTER 4
CHAMPAGNE AND OYSTERS

*A*h … champagne and oysters. Luxury … romance … can life get any better than this? Well, actually, yes. Add yoga to this extravagance and your evening will become a new, complete—and, soon, essential—delight.

RECIPE FOR EXTRAVAGANCE:

1 PART TREATING YOURSELF
1 PART BUBBLES
2 PARTS UNIVERSAL ACCEPTANCE
GARNISH WITH CONSCIOUS BREATHING

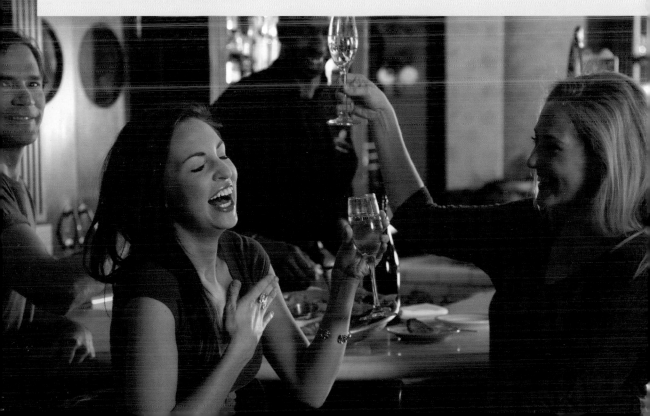

Whiskey Wower

So why is Jenna so "wowed" in the photo on the right? It must be because Sara actually has her heel down in this variation of Warrior I. Keeping the back heel down while keeping the front hip bones aligned is extremely difficult, even for the most flexible yogi or yogini. Try the version Sara is doing, which helps stabilize the lower torso or try the classical pose below. And whether you're wearing heels or not, work on keeping your back heel down.

WHAT YOU DO

1. Use a low bar stool or bar chair. This helps you keep your sternum, lower back, and lower abs lifted throughout the pose.

2. Stand facing the back of the chair, with your feet approximately 3 ½ to 4 feet apart.

3. Place your hands on the back of the chair.

4. Attempting to keep your front hip bones even and your back heel down, slowly bend your forward leg into a right angle (or close to a right angle).

5. Hold for 60 seconds, release, and switch sides.

Benefits: This pose helps build strength in the legs, lower back, and lower abdomen. It increases flexibility in the hips and shoulders.

For the traditional pose, follow the same basic instructions, but without the chair. Lift your arms overhead, with your elbows straight and your palms facing each other.

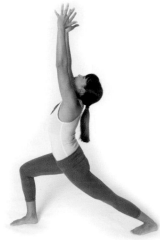

Happy Hour Hint

If you cannot keep your heel down and your front hip bones aligned, place your back heel on a wall, 2 to 3 inches from the floor and press your heel firmly into the wall. Practice this pose along with other standing poses throughout the book for the full range of strengthening benefits.

Ask Your Bartender For . . .

A Whiskey Sour, with whiskey, lemon juice, sugar, and a cherry on top.

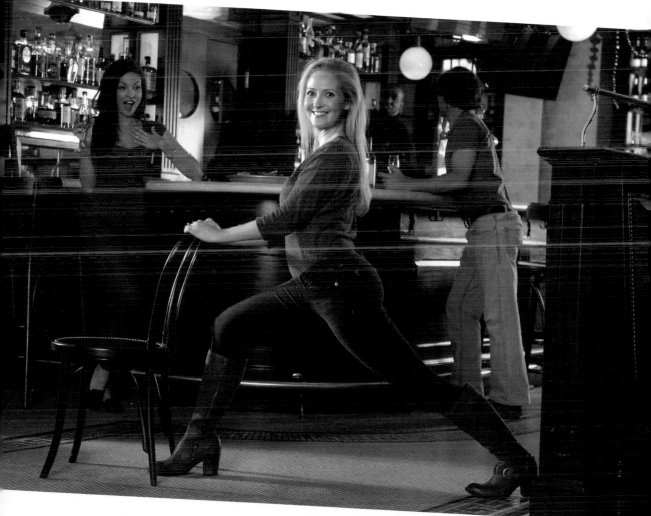

Wobbly Warrior

Everyone who has practiced this pose knows that Wobbly Warrior is an appropriate name. It is a little tricky to get into, it is difficult to hold the balance and the alignment, and most of us do not come out of the pose gracefully—sort of like getting in and out of a cab on a Friday night. It is a very challenging pose—even without champagne. Note: Traditionally known as Warrior III, this pose is an extension of Warrior I pose. However, we will cheat a little to make it easier.

WHAT YOU DO

1. Align two bar stools so that the distance between them is the full length of your body with your arms extended.

2. Place your forearms on the seat of one bar stool.

3. Walk backwards until your torso and legs form a right angle.

4. Lift one leg and place it on the stool behind you.

5. Have a friend help make sure that your front hip bones are even.

6. Hold for 60 seconds or longer. Release and switch sides.

Benefits: Builds strength and flexibility in the thighs, hips, torso, and shoulders. Increases ability to balance.

For home practice, start in Warrior I pose (page 56), and then lean forward, bringing your torso over your front thigh. Pause for a moment. Straighten your front leg and bring your back leg up, aligning it with your hips. Strongly extend your arms in front of you and your back leg behind you.

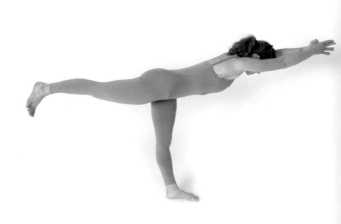

If you're a beginner, keep your head in line with your spine. Once you've gotten some practice with this pose, work on looking out past your hands.

Ask Your Bartender For . . .

A Wobbly Knee, with amaretto, coffee liqueur, vodka, coconut cream, and double cream.

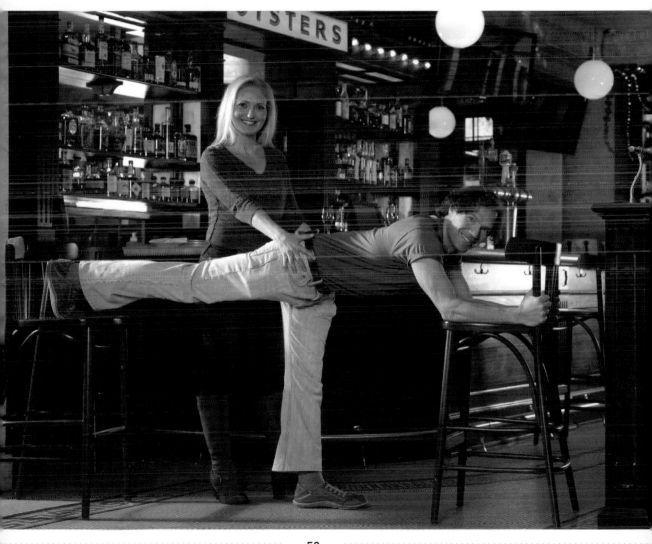

Blue Moon

In Sanskrit, this pose is called Ardha Chandrasana, or Half Moon pose. The pose is graceful and elegant, and mastering it will help you embody these wonderful qualities. We have renamed it Blue Moon pose, and in practicing this pose regularly, you will feel like a Moon Goddess or maybe the Man on the Moon. Later, enjoy a Blue Moon cocktail or some Blue Point oysters.

WHAT YOU DO

1. Align two bar stools (preferably with backs) approximately your height apart.

2. Turn your forward foot toward the chair.

3. Place your forward hand on one of the bar stool rungs and the side of your foot on the top of the other bar stool. Adjust to make sure that each foot is aligned with your hip.

4. Have a friend help you rotate your torso backwards. And, try to roll your thighs outward.

5. Keep your head aligned with your spine, otherwise your neck will ache later.

6. Hold for 60 seconds. Slowly release and switch sides.

Benefits: Strengthens and increases flexibility in the legs, torso, shoulders, and arms. Improves your ability to balance and your self-confidence.

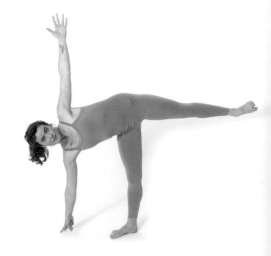

When practicing at home, remember that this is an extension of Side Angle pose (page 62). From Side Angle pose, straighten your forward leg while lifting your back leg. Place your hand on the floor or on a yoga block. Firmly extend your right leg behind you. Slightly rotate your torso backward. Gently release and switch sides.

Happy Hour Hint

To help balance, you can practice this pose with your back foot on the wall. Your starting stance will have to be a little narrower, and you may have to practice a few times before you get it right. Once there, firmly press your foot into the wall. Having your foot on the wall will also help you rotate your torso and roll your thigh muscles outward.

Ask Your Bartender For . . .

A Blue Moon, which includes gin, curacao liqueur, sweet and sour mix, and pineapple juice.

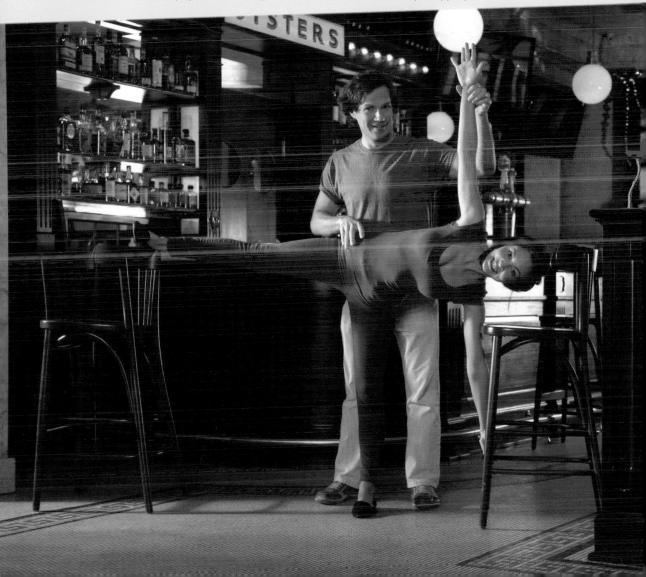

Bay Breeze

This pose is traditionally called Extended Side Angle pose. Yet despite its clinical name, it is an enjoyable pose that helps people feel light. The Bay Breeze cocktail is also light … and breezy … and after a few of them, you'll be breezy, too.

WHAT YOU DO

1. It is best to use bar chairs, or very short bar stools for this pose.

2. Start with your feet 4 to 4 ½ feet wide, facing forward.

3. Turn your right foot out 90 degrees and your left foot in about 15 degrees.

4. Extend your arms to the side, shoulder height and stretch evenly from your shoulders to your fingertips.

5. Slowly bend your forward leg into a Right Angle (see Warrior II on page 20).

6. With your torso facing forward, move from your hip crease and intensely stretch the right side of your torso over the top of your thigh. Bring your right hand to the seat of the bar chair or the rung of a bar stool.

7. Bring your left arm over your ear and extend your arm as though you are extending it from your left foot through your fingertips.

8. Hold this pose for about 60 seconds. Release slowly, first coming back into Warrior II pose, and then standing up. Switch sides.

Benefits: Increases flexibility in the legs, torso, shoulders, and arms. Also builds strength in the arms and hips.

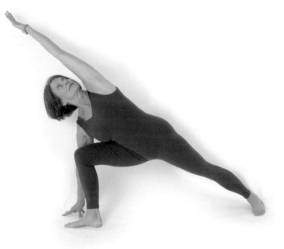

For home practice, start in the same manner as the bar stool pose. Place your hand on the floor or on a yoga block. Stretch from your foot to your fingertips. Press your thigh into your arm and your arm into your thigh.

Happy Hour Hint

To increase your stretch and stability in the pose, place the side of your back foot at a wall and firmly press it into the wall.

Ask Your Bartender For . . .

A Bay Breeze, with cranberry juice, pineapple juice, and vodka.

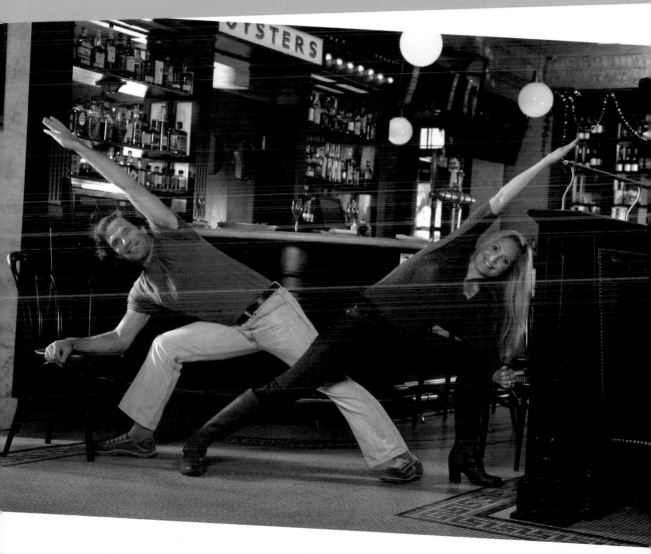

Angel Face

This is a variation of Intense Chest Stretch pose. The Angel Face cocktail is an apple brandy-based drink from France. Looking at Sara doing this pose, you can tell why we renamed it.

WHAT YOU DO

1. Stand in front of a short bar stool, about 2 feet from the seat.

2. Walk one foot forward so the foot is under the seat, and walk the other foot back about 1 foot. Remember to align properly.

3. Bend forward from your hip crease and keep your spine extended. Place your hands on the seat of the bar stool.

4. Continue to stretch your spine, leading with your sternum. Keep your front hipbones even. Keep your head in line with your torso.

5. Hold for 60 to 90 seconds. Slowly come up and switch sides.

Benefits: This pose stretches and strengthens the back muscles and increases flexibility in your hamstrings.

The traditional pose directions are identical to the bar stool pose, except that you place your hands on yoga blocks.

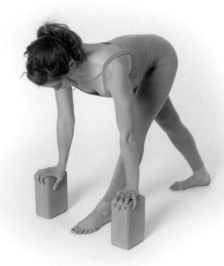

Happy Hour Hint

As you advance in the pose, you can slide your chest down your leg and, eventually, bring your hands to the floor.

Ask Your Bartender For . . .

An Angel Face with apple brandy, apricot brandy, and gin.

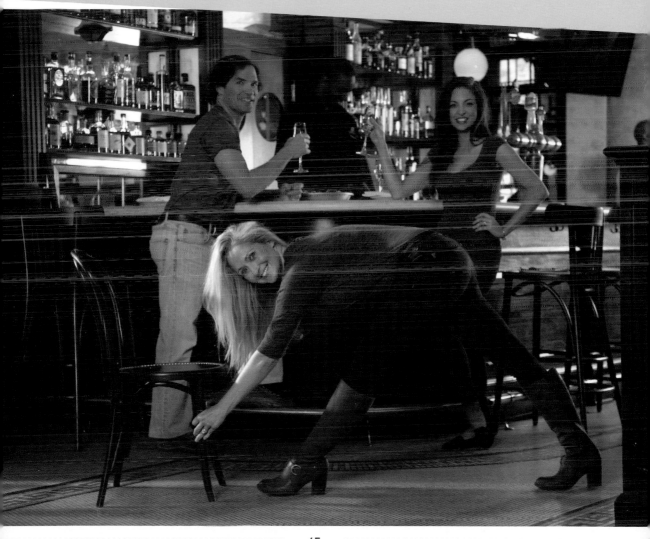

Latin Twist

We recently discovered a new champagne cocktail, complete with acai berry liqueur, blueberries, and a twist of your favorite citrus. Today's favorite twist is the Revolved Triangle, which will enhance your strength, flexibility, and balance. And, in this case, your balance will improve if you are on (or rather using) a bar stool.

WHAT YOU DO

1. Stand with your feet 3 ½ to 4 feet apart, facing forward.

2. Rotate your torso to the left until the front of your torso completely faces your forward leg. Engage your quadriceps. Rotate your forward thigh outward and your back thigh inward.

3. Firmly press your back heel into the floor.

4. Extend your left arm and your torso forward. Rotate your torso to the right (backwards). Place your right palm on the seat of the bar stool and your left palm on your hip.

5. Continue to engage your thighs and rotate the forward thigh outward and the back thigh inward. At the same time, press the front of your thighs to the back of your thighs.

6. On each inhalation, lengthen your spine a little bit more, and on each exhalation, twist farther to the right. The twist originates from the very bottom of your spine.

7. Hold for about 60 seconds. Unwind on an inhalation and repeat the pose on the other side.

Benefits: This pose will increase flexibility, balance, and strength.

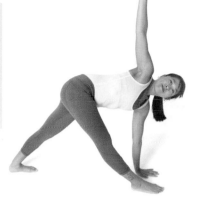

The traditional pose differs in that you place your hand on the floor or on a yoga block. You can place your hand in front of your foot or behind it, depending on your flexibility in the pose. If your heel automatically lifts up, place your heel on the wall and firmly press it into it.

Happy Hour Hint

Ideally your hand and prop will be on the outside of your forward leg, but some yoga students are aligned more appropriately if their hand is on the inside of the forward leg.

Ask Your Bartender For . . .

A Latin Twist with acai berry liqueur, champagne, and a blueberry or two for garnish.

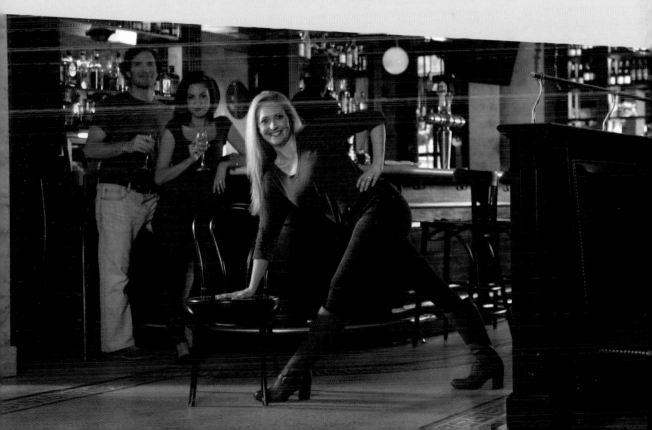

Kir Royale

You're always bending over backwards for your friends. Now you can bend over backwards *with* your friends. There are many ways to practice backbends, both passively and actively. They are fun, exhilarating, and in doing them, we further open our hearts to both old and new friends.

WHAT YOU DO

1. Stand behind a low bar stool. Have one friend in front of you and the other friend behind you.

2. Have one friend hold your lower back and help you drop back over the top of the bar stool back. Your lower back should be on the bar stool and the crown of your head should be parallel to the floor.

3. Reach out and take hold of your other friend's waist. She will hold your forearms.

4. Hold for 30 to 60 seconds. When you release, have your friend who is holding your lower back hold it very firmly as he helps lift you.

5. Bring your head up last and rest for a moment so you do not get dizzy.

6. Then let one of your other friends take a turn.

Benefits: Increases flexibility in the back, legs, shoulders, arms, and spine.

To practice at home with a chair, slide your hips so they are on the edge of the seat. Lean backwards, placing the middle of your back on the seat edge and your hands on the floor, fingers facing you. Keep your forearms parallel. Breathe! When you come up, hold the sides of the chair. Bring your head up last. Lean forward for a few moments to prevent dizziness.

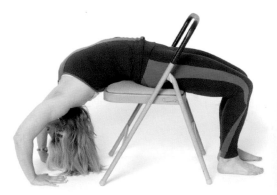

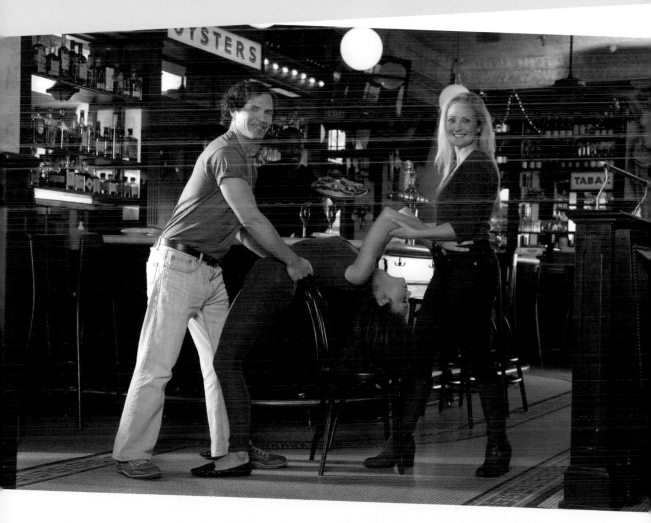

CHAPTER 5
FLIRTINI NIGHT

The bar for impressing your girl has just gotten a whole lot higher. How can the average guy possibly compete with headstands on the bar (especially if the girl is a Martini Yogini)? No more "What do you do?" Or "Who did your tattoo?" The new normal is "How are your arm balances?" and "Show me your Warrior pose." Forget the fancy cars, forget the six-pack abs (um, never mind, don't forget the abs), girls want to see your Chaturanga Dandasana. So, sorry dancing-on-the-bar dude, today's man flirts by impressing his date with his balance and equanimity (and yoga abs).

RECIPE FOR FLIRTINI*:

1 PART BALANCE
2 PARTS POISE
6 PARTS ABS
1 PART INNER PEACE
GARNISH WITH ONE-POINTED ATTENTION TO YOUR POSE

* The real Flirtini cocktail was developed for *Sex and the City* actress Sarah Jessica Parker by a bartender at Guastavino's in New York City. This is a pink, fruity, bubbly drink that does not have a strong alcoholic taste. It is easy to over-indulge with this fun concoction, so be careful.

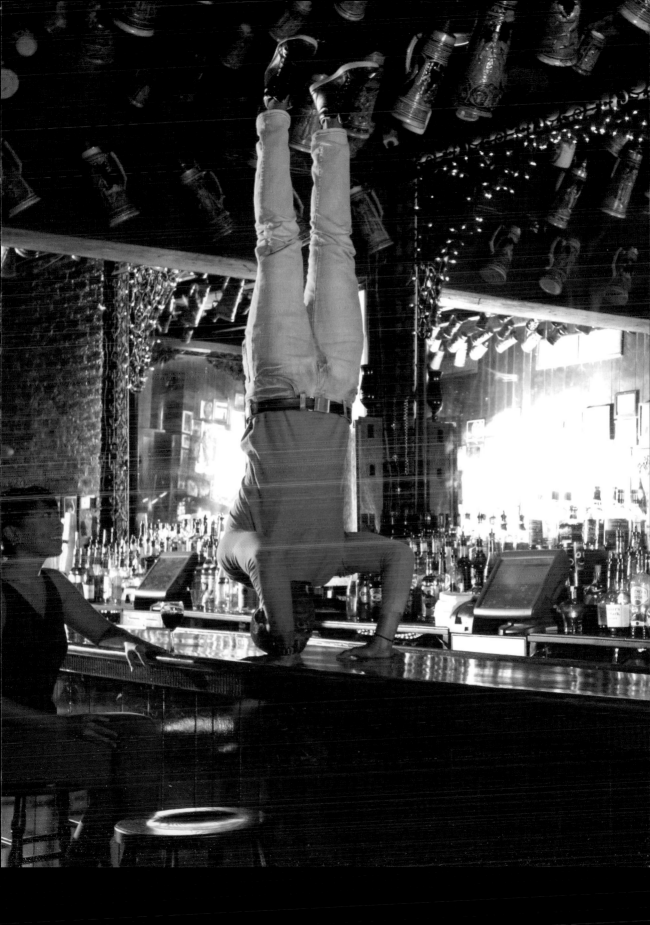

Sidecar

Guys aren't the only ones who get to show off their yoga prowess. Jimmy is clearly impressed as Ananda effortlessly demonstrates one of the most difficult arm balances ... on a bar stool! This pose is traditionally called Eight-Angle pose, yet it is reminiscent of the sidecar of a motorcycle, for which the famous drink was named during World War I in Paris. Have fun doing Sidecar with a friend.

WHAT YOU DO

1. For this pose, we are giving the directions for practicing it on the floor or on a bar. This is a very advanced pose and should only be attempted on the bar stool if you truly have mastered this pose on the floor first.

2. Start by standing with your feet about 18 inches apart. Bend your knees, rest your right palm on the floor between your feet, and place your left palm on the floor, on the outside of your left foot.

3. Bring your right leg over your right arm and rest the back of your right thigh on the back of your right arm, just below your elbow. Bring your left leg forward between your arms, but closer to your right arm.

4. Exhale and lift both of your legs off the floor. Interlock the legs by placing the left foot upon the right at the ankle and extend your legs sideways to the right. Your right arm will be gripped between the thighs and will be slightly bent at the elbow. Your left arm should be straight.

5. On an exhalation, bend your elbows and lower your torso and head until they are parallel with the floor. Hold, breathing evenly, and, if you are so inclined, move your head and torso from side to side.

6. Hold as long as you like. To release: straighten your arms, raise your torso, uncross your legs and lower them to the floor.

7. Repeat on the other side.

Benefits: Strengthens the wrists, arms, and shoulders, tones the abdominals and inner thighs, and improves balance.

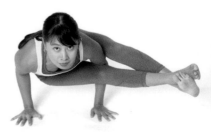

Do not attempt this advanced pose on a bar stool until you have mastered it first on the floor or on a mat.

Happy Hour Hint

If you decide to use a bar stool, make sure it is stable, and have a friend hold it, if necessary. Plus, have an extra stool or two available to help you get into the pose. Then have a friend pull the extra stools out of the way.

Ask Your Bartender For . . .

A Sidecar, which consists of triple sec, cognac, and lemon juice.

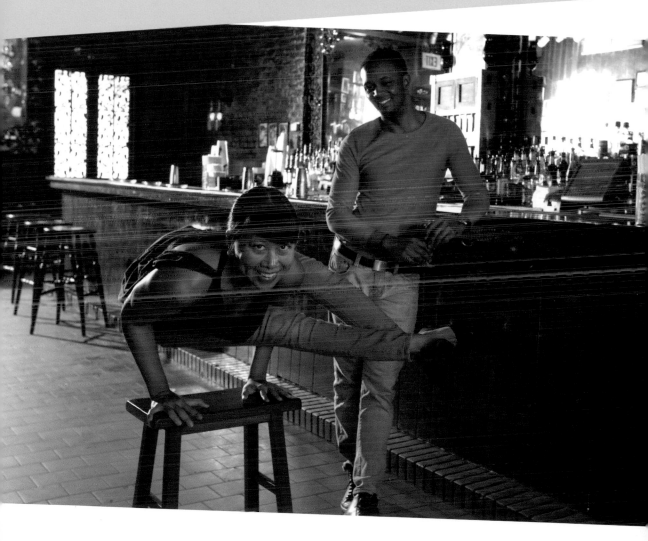

Canadian Cranes and Caesars

This pose resembles a crane and, thus, that is its name. Many years ago, Canadian cranes migrated each winter to a field near my home, so I have particular fondness for Canadian cranes. Watch out: These yoga birds may take flight … to get at Canada's most popular drink, the Canadian Caesar.

WHAT YOU DO

1. For this pose, we are giving directions for on a bar or the floor. This is a very advanced pose and should only be attempted on a bar stool once you have truly mastered it on the floor.

2. Stand with your feet a little wider than your hips. Squat, bend your elbows, and place your palms on the floor. Place the backs of your upper arms against your shins.

3. Take a few moments to maneuver your inner thighs against the sides of your torso and your shins into your armpits. Slide your upper arms as low as possible onto your shins.

4. Lift your heels and lean forward, placing your weight on the backs of your upper arms. Contract your abs and round your back. With a very subtle movement, allow your tailbone to drop toward the floor.

5. Lean forward onto your upper arms until your feet are off the floor.

6. Now, on an exhalation, lean further forward onto your upper arms until your feet are off the floor.

7. Now that you are balanced on the back of your legs, assertively squeeze your legs against your arms, press your hands firmly into the floor, and straighten your elbows.

8. Keep your head in line with your spine, or looking down slightly.

9. Stay in the pose as long as you like and release by bending your elbows and bringing your feet back to the floor, into a squat position.

Benefits: Builds strength in your arms, shoulders, and abs.

Happy Hour Hint

If you decide to use a bar stool, make sure it is stable, and have a friend hold it, if necessary. Plus, have an extra stool or two available to help you get into the pose. Then have a friend pull the stools out when your photo is being snapped.

Ask Your Bartender For . . .

The Caesar or Canadian Caesar was invented in 1969 by restaurant manager Walter Chell of the Calgary Inn in Calgary, Alberta, Canada. He devised the cocktail after being asked to create a signature drink for the Calgary Inn's new Italian restaurant. It is a mixture of vodka, clam juice, tomato juice, and other spices. Chell was of Italian descent and he reasoned that in Venice he had had spaghetti with a vodka, tomato, and clam sauce. The popularity of the drink skyrocketed and became Canada's most popular drink.

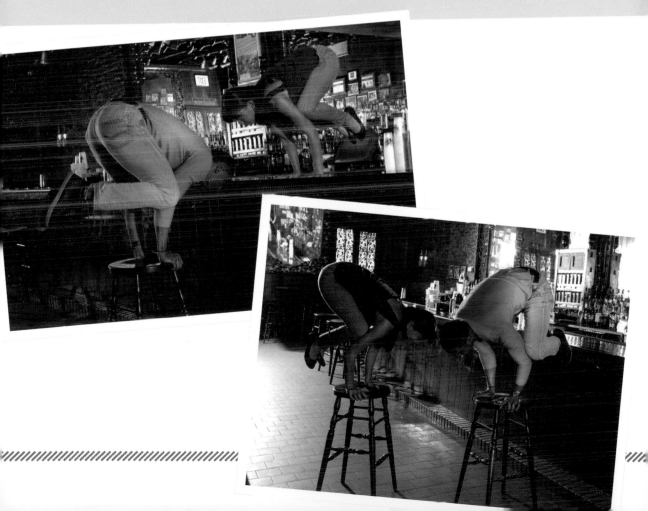

Hurricane

Called Bow pose in yoga, it resembles what a hurricane looks like on a weather map. But this hurricane is beneficial, not destructive, even if you are practicing in a crowded bar.

WHAT YOU DO

1. As in the previous two poses, if you are using a bar stool, make sure it is stable and have a friend hold it, if necessary.

2. Place your abdomen and hip bones on the bar stool.

3. Lift your legs up behind you, as high as you can.

4. Reach back and grasp your ankles with your hands. Lift your legs and your chest as high as possible. As you lift your chest, bring your upper back in toward your chest.

5. Bring your head back. Hold the pose as long as you like. Release, rest for a few moments, and try again.

Benefits: This pose stretches the spine, shoulders, and arms.

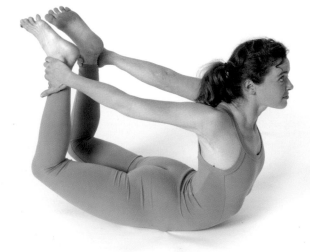

Classically, this pose is done with only the abdomen on the floor and the legs together. However, beginner and intermediate students should have their hip bones and top of their thighs on the floor, as well.

Happy Hour Hint

Breathe evenly and deliberately, as breathing in this pose can be somewhat difficult.

Ask Your Bartender For . . .

A Hurricane, which was first created in the mid-1940s at the world famous Pat O'Brien's bar in the French Quarter of New Orleans. During this time, there was a shortage of bourbon and scotch. So the liquor salesmen had to convince bar owners to buy very large quantities of rum, which was unpopular and difficult to sell. If a bar owner bought 50 or more cases of rum, they could then buy the bourbon and scotch that they really wanted. Through trial and error, Pat O'Brien, one of the owners, created a drink with four ounces of a booze nobody wanted, with lemon juice, passion fruit syrup, and crushed ice and put it in a glass that looked like a hurricane lamp. The drink and the bar's business exploded and made the bar a legend. Lucky for us, we were able to photograph this pose at Pat O'Brien's!

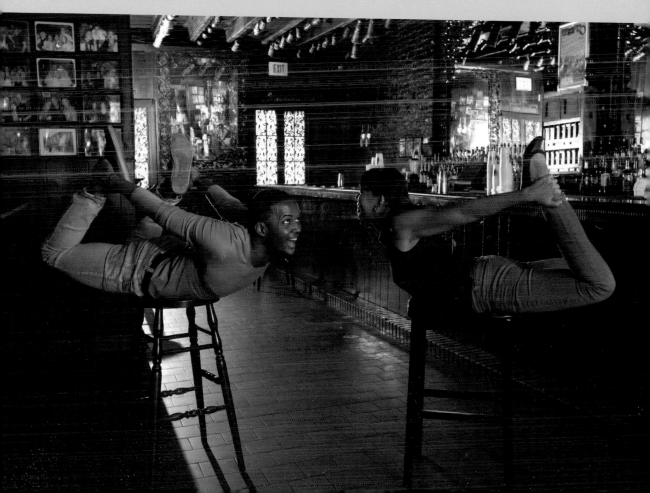

Peaceful Warrior

Here's another Warrior pose, which verges on acrobatic yoga if done on bar stools. Not the greatest pose for a crowded Friday night at the bar; yet feeling like a Peaceful Warrior after a long week of work is wonderful.

WHAT YOU DO

1. Align two bar stools, approximately 4 feet apart. Carefully climb on the bar stools, with one foot on each. Make sure the bar stools are stable and have friends hold them if necessary.

2. Turn your right foot out 90 degrees and turn your left foot inward approximately 15 degrees, aligning the heel of your right foot with the arch of your back foot.

3. Extend your arms fully, aligning your hands with your shoulders. Relax the top of your shoulders.

4. Bend your right (forward) knee into a right angle.

5. Bring your left hand behind your back. Gently shift your torso toward your back leg.

6. Lift your right arm straight up and gaze at your hand.

7. Hold for 45 to 60 seconds. Slowly release and repeat on the other side.

Benefits: Builds strength in the legs and lower back and increases flexibility in the arms and shoulders.

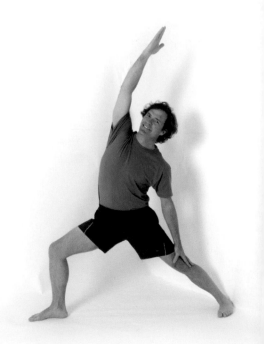

Another version of this pose is to slide your back hand down your leg and to reach your forward hand toward your back foot.

Happy Hour Hint

If you feel any compression in your spine when bringing your forward arm behind you, bring your arm forward again.

Ask Your Bartender For . . .

A World Peace, which was created by master mixologist Jonathan Pogash for the World Bar, which is opposite the United Nations in New York. This blue cocktail includes gin, elderflower syrup, blue curacao, almond syrup, and lemon juice. If you visit the World Bar and order this drink, 15-percent of the price will be donated to UN peacekeeping efforts.

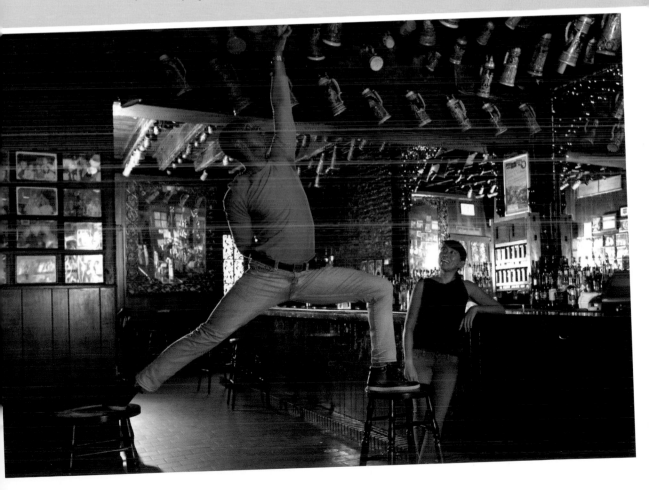

Cable Car

This cool-looking, and not-so-easy posture is called Bound Side Angle pose. In looking at the pose, it reminds me of a rail car … or maybe a cable car. The cocktail was created in 1996 as a signature drink at the Starlight Room, an elegant cocktail bar at the top of the Sir Francis Drake Hotel in San Francisco. The drink commemorates the city's famous cable car. And maybe, just maybe … with some imagination, the bar stools resemble cable car tracks.

WHAT YOU DO

1. Align two bar stools, approximately 4 feet apart. Carefully climb on the bar stools, with one foot on each. Make sure the stools are stable and have friends hold them if necessary.

2. Turn your left foot out 90 degrees and turn your right foot inward approximately 15 degrees, aligning the heel of your left foot with the arch of your right foot.

3. Extend your arms fully, aligning your hands with your shoulders. Relax the top of your shoulders.

4. Bend your left knee into a right angle. Moving from your hip crease, extend the side of your torso over your left thigh.

5. Bring your right arm behind you and your left arm beneath your thigh and behind your back, clasping your hands.

6. Rotate your torso toward the wall behind you.

7. Breathe evenly and hold for 30 to 60 seconds. Gently release by coming back into Side Angle pose (page 62), and then Warrior II (page 20), and finally back to standing. Repeat on the other side.

8. Carefully come down from the bar stools, perhaps with a friend's help.

Benefits: Strengthens legs and abs, and increases flexibility in the arms and shoulders.

Practicing on the floor is the same as the bar stool pose, without the fear of falling.

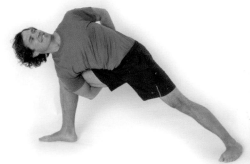

Happy Hour Hint

If you cannot clasp your hands behind your back, practice with a yoga strap or old necktie between your hands. The strap will give you more room to work into the pose.

Ask Your Bartender For . . .

A Cable Car, which contains orange curacao, spiced rum, lime juice, and sweet and sour mix.

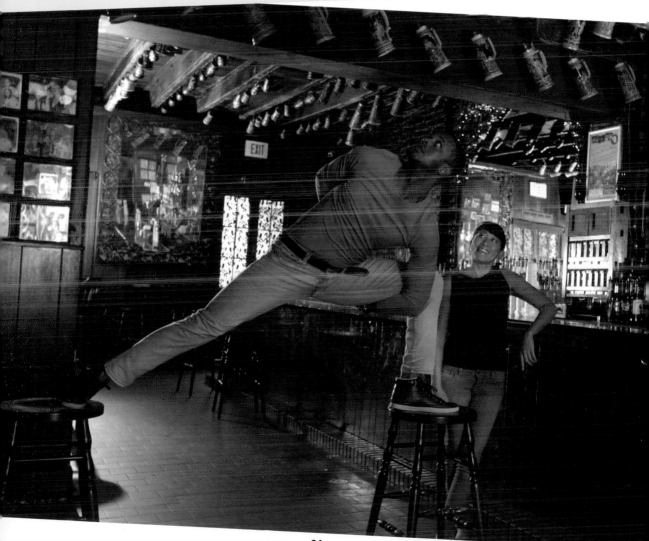

Daiquiri Dance

Normally called Dancer's pose, this advanced backbend should normally be done only after a vigorous practice of standing poses and backbends. Attempting this pose before one is truly ready for such an intense backbend can compress the lower back. Placing your thigh on a bar stool helps beginner and intermediate students safely practice this pose before they are ready for the full pose. The photos and the instructions here are modified for those just beginning to attempt this beautiful pose.

WHAT YOU DO

1. Stand in front of a bar stool with your feet together, your thighs engaged, your lower back and lower abdomen lifted, your sternum lifted, and your shoulders, neck, and throat relaxed.

2. Shift your weight to your left leg. Lift your right leg behind you and place your thigh on the bar stool.

3. Reach back with your right hand and clasp the outside of your foot or ankle.

4. Continually lift your sternum and your lower abdomen upward. Actively move your lower back and tailbone inward, toward your abdomen. These movements protect the lower back and are more easily mastered with your thigh on the bar stool.

5. Stay in the pose as long as you like. To release, come back to standing by letting go of your foot and bringing your leg down and your torso up. Repeat on the other side.

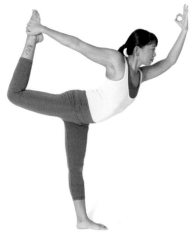

Benefits: This graceful pose enhances flexibility and develops balance and poise.

When practicing this pose without the bar stool, over time you can lift your chest and your leg higher. Be sure to use the alignment instructions for your sternum, lower abdomen, and lower back detailed in the bar stool pose.

In addition to having practiced standing poses and other backbends before attempting this pose, also make sure your quadriceps and psoas muscles are warmed up and stretched.

Ask Your Bartender For...

A Daiquiri, which was supposedly created in the beach and mining town of Daiquiri, Cuba in the early 1900s. The story goes that a U.S. mining engineer who was working there, Jennings Cox, ran out of gin at a party. So, he decided to blend rum, sugar cane, and limes together. In 1909, a U.S. Navy doctor discovered the drink while in Cuba and brought the recipe to the Army and Navy Club in Washington, D.C. Popularity of the drink spread after F. Scott Fitzgerald mentioned the Daiquiri in his book, *This Side of Paradise*, which was published in 1920. The drink, and other rum-based drinks, became more popular during World War II, when war rationing made gin, scotch, and bourbon difficult to get. At that time, trade was increased with Latin America, and rum was easy to get. Daiquiris are so popular in the U.S. that National Daiquiri Day is celebrated each year on July 19th.

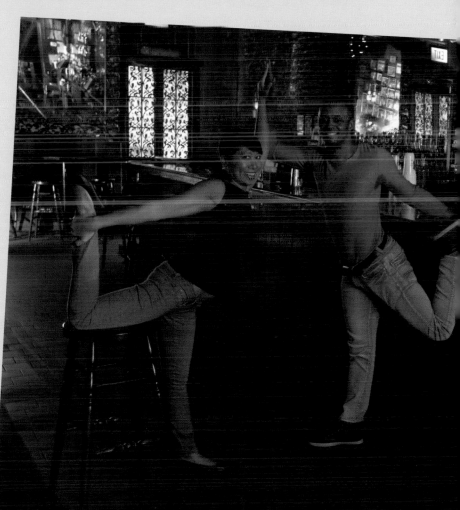

Night Cap

In India, the traditional hello and goodbye greeting is a bow, with hands at the heart or near the face. At the end of most yoga classes, the teacher and the students bow to each other. The gesture is called Namaskar and is a recognition that there is a spark of divinity in everyone. The bow acknowledges and reveres that divinity. The greeting they voice is "namaste," which means "I bow to you." It can also mean, "The Divine in me honors the Divine in you." The gesture is deeply heartfelt, one that expresses gratitude and oneness. If you feel a sense of gratitude for (and oneness with) your date, perhaps this gesture is appropriate at the end of a fun evening.

WHAT YOU DO

1. Sit on a bar stool, with your legs crossed, facing your date. Place your hands at your heart.

2. Remind yourself of your connection and your date's connection to the Divine, your oneness with God (or any other name you may use for God: Universal Reality, Cosmic Conscious, etc.).

3. Lean forward and bow to that spark of Divinity within him or her.

The pose is the same, whether you are sitting on the floor or on a bar stool.

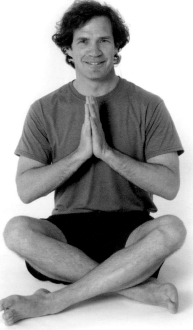

Happy Hour Hint

No matter where you are or who you are with, you can always bow to the divinity in others, even if you only do this in your heart, without the posture.

Ask Your Bartender For . . .

A Nightcap, which includes coffee liqueur, nutmeg, milk, and powdered sugar.

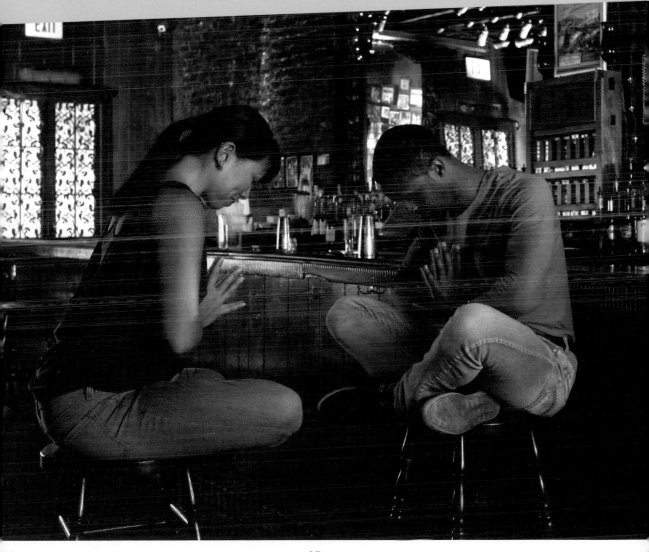

CHAPTER 6
PUTTIN' ON THE RITZ

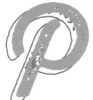erhaps the song says it best: "…Spending every dime on a wonderful time." However, even if you don't have too many dimes to spend, there's something simply splendid about dressing up in your finest for a wonderful night on the town. Just remember, whether white tie or black tie, formal or informal, getting gussied up doesn't have to mean forgoing your newfound love for bar stool yoga. Even in your finest formal eveningwear, you can twist, turn, bend, and breathe. Think of it as being expansive even when the clothing is expensive.

RECIPE FOR FEELING GLITZY:

1 PART EVENINGWEAR

1 PART JEWELRY

1 PART STIFF SHIRT AND BOW TIE

1 PART FAVORITE DANCE PARTNER OR
 WEDDING DATE

2 PARTS OPEN BAR

GARNISH WITH SILLINESS

SERVE ON SPECIAL OCCASIONS

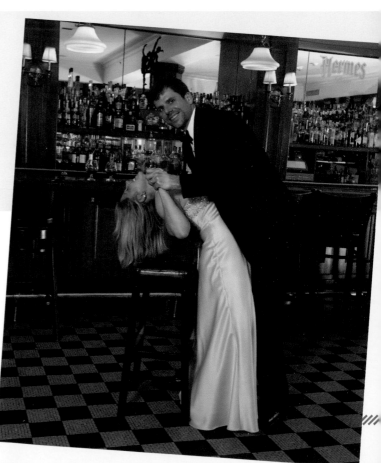

Old Fashioned

Dressing up to go out on the town? Maybe that is a little old fashioned these days, but it sure looks like fun, especially when doing an old-fashioned yoga posture like Extended Hand to Toe pose. Not sure which is older, the yoga pose or the cocktail.

WHAT YOU DO

1. Stand with your feet together. Shift your weight to one leg. Bend and lift your opposite leg and place your foot on the bar stool. (See photo on next page.)

2. Lean forward and clasp your partner's hands. Gently pull him or her toward you, and smile.

3. Hold as long as you wish. Release and switch sides.

Benefits: Increases flexibility in the hamstrings and strength in the lower back.

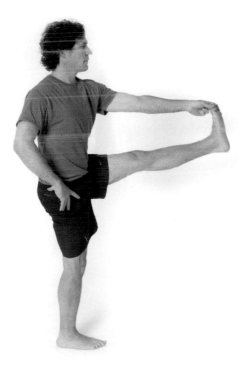

For at-home practice, when you lift your leg, clasp the outside of your foot or your big toe and then extend your leg forward. Straighten both knees. Hold for 30 to 60 seconds. Lower your foot to the floor. Repeat on the other side.

If your hamstrings are tight, hold a strap or old necktie looped around your extended foot.

Ask Your Bartender For . . .

An Old Fashioned, which includes bourbon, bitters, water, sugar, a maraschino cherry, and an orange wedge. There are various accounts of how the Old Fashioned cocktail was invented. Its recipe and origin were mentioned in the *Chicago Daily Tribune* in the early 1880s, and a recipe from seventy-five years earlier is mentioned in the article. This cocktail truly is old fashioned.

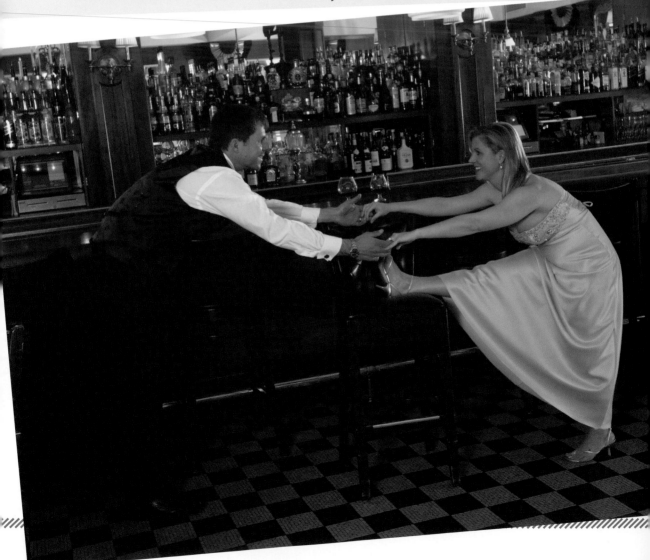

Mint Julep

What a beautiful, graceful pose! It's called Revolved Utthita Padagustanasana or Revolved Hand to Foot pose. This version is a lot more fun than the traditional pose because you get to hold your partner's hand rather than your own foot. This pose must go with Mint Juleps, which though has its origin in London, is considered the classic drink of the American South.

WHAT YOU DO

1. Stand with your feet hip distance apart. Follow the detailed alignment instructions on page 8.

2. Bend your left leg and place your heel on the bar stool. Place your left hand on your hip. Your partner will use the right leg. (See photo on next page.)

3. Gently twist your torso toward your left leg, twisting from the very bottom of your spine.

4. Hold your partner's hand and smile.

5. Hold as long as you like. Release and switch sides.

Benefits: Increases strength and flexibility in your legs and hips. Enhances balance and poise.

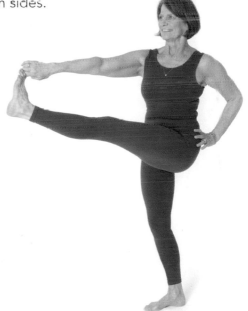

For the traditional pose, lift your left leg, and clasp your big toe with your right hand. Extend your left leg forward while straightening your right arm. Turn your torso toward your left leg. Work on keeping both legs straight and your torso lifted.

Happy Hour Hint

When practicing alone, if your hand does not quite reach your foot, place a yoga strap or necktie around your extended foot and hold both ends of the strap in your opposite hand.

Ask Your Bartender For . . .

A Mint Julep, which includes bourbon, powdered sugar, water, and fresh mint sprigs.

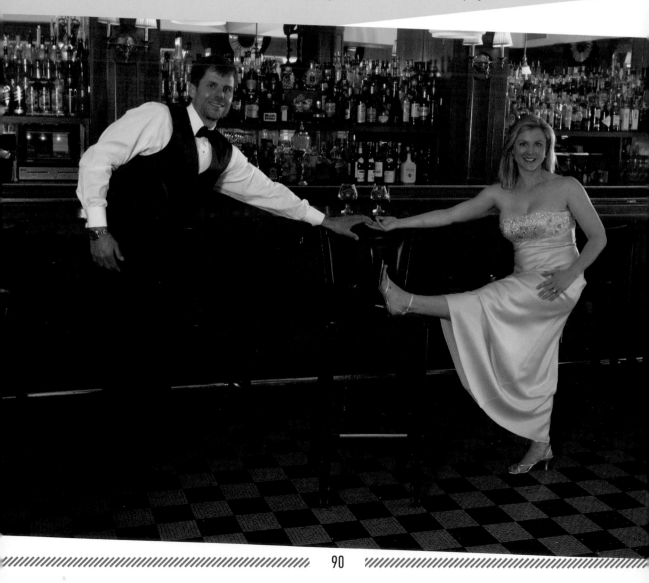

French Connection

Paschimottanasana, or Intense West pose, is normally done alone; however, working with a partner on bar stools can be both beneficial and fun. Made of cognac and amaretto, a French Connection is an exquisite after-dinner drink, and the perfect name for this pose if you are working with a partner.

WHAT YOU DO

1. With your partner, sit on bar stools with a bar stool between you. (See photo on next page.)

2. Place your heels on the middle bar stool.

3. Bend forward from your hip crease. Extend from the base of your spine and as evenly as possible extend your sternum toward your feet.

4. Hold your partner's hands and gently pull toward yourselves.

5. Stay in the pose as long as you like, enjoying each other's company.

6. You can also take turns gently pulling each other forward firmly and evenly so your spine and back muscles are extended as much as possible.

Benefits: Stretches the hamstrings and the back. Great way to connect with your date.

Allow your body to gradually release rather than forcing further extension. If you cannot touch your toes, place your hands on your knees, shins, or ankles.

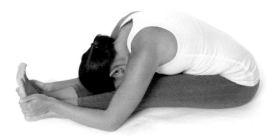

Happy Hour Hint

While engaging your quadriceps, try rolling your thighs inward and pressing your thighs firmly toward the floor. This allows your spine to extend more completely.

Ask Your Bartender For . . .

A French Connection, which is a combination of cognac and amaretto.

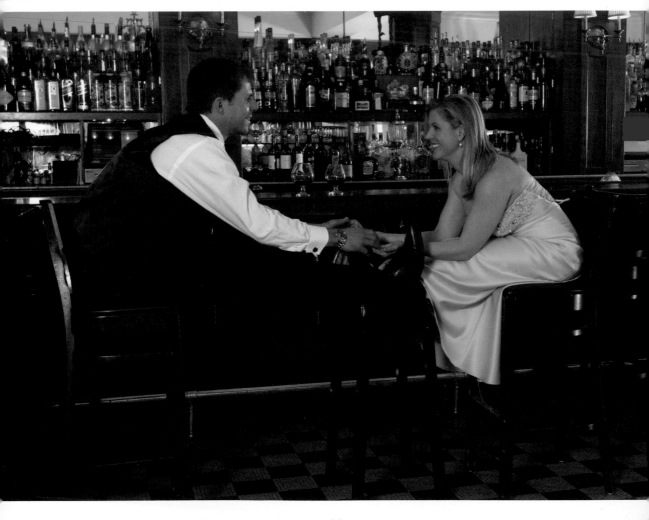

Lady of Leisure

This is truly a very sophisticated, graceful, pose ... perhaps one that only a lady of leisure has time to master. This pose, Hanumanasana, is named after a monkey god in Hindu mythology, Hanuman. In one of the ancient Hindu stories, Hanuman jumps across India several times to save the life of a goddess. This pose imitates how wide his legs must have been jumping across land and sea, thus the origin of the Sanskrit name of what we normally call a Full Split.

WHAT YOU DO

1. This is an advanced pose, hence it is described here with props to get you started.

2. Kneeling on the bar, bring one foot in front of you, as in a Lunge pose (page 7). Place one or two yoga blocks under your torso and hide them with your long dress. (See photo on next page.)

3. Carefully slide your feet away from each other, until you are on the blocks.

4. Place your hands in prayer position at your heart and smile at your partner.

5. Hold as long as you like. Release (maybe with your partner's help) and switch legs.

Benefits: This pose intensely stretches the legs and psoas muscles.

At home, you will need a slick surface for this pose. Place a bolster on the floor and two yoga blocks in front of the bolster. Come into a Lunge pose (see page 7), and place your hands on the blocks. Slide your feet away from each other. Keep your torso over your hips.

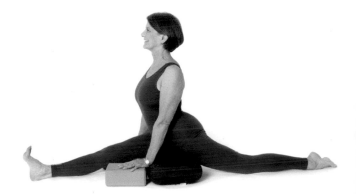

Be sure to warm up your hamstrings, quadriceps, psoas muscles, and hips prior to attempting this pose. And definitely use the props to get started.

Ask Your Bartender For . . .

A Lady of Leisure cocktail, which is served primarily in England. Its ingredients are gin, pineapple juice, raspberry liqueur, triple sec, and orange.

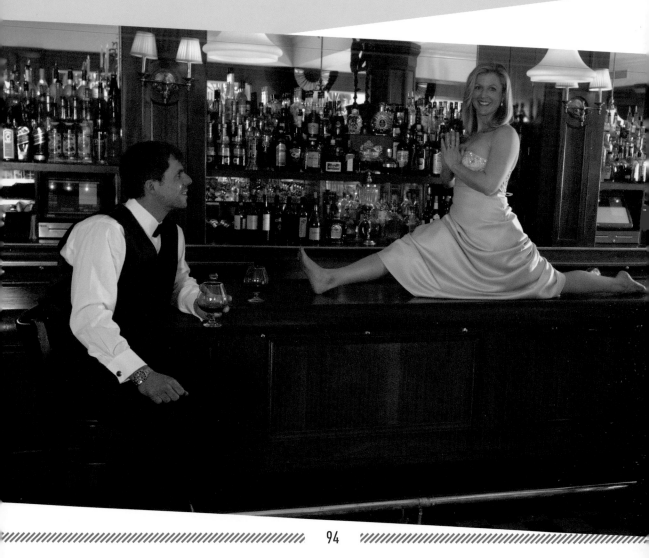

Cosmopolitan

The elegance, grace, and sophistication of a backbend, particularly in a lovely evening gown. Definitely a Cosmopolitan look, wouldn't you agree?

WHAT YOU DO

1. Place a bar stool, preferably with a padded seat, a few inches behind you. Make sure that it is stable. (See photo on next page.)

2. With your legs hip-width apart and your thighs rolling toward each other, bend your knees. Have your date help you slowly bend backwards until your back is on the seat of the bar stool.

3. Allow your head to drop completely.

4. You can hold the bar stool or your date's hand, or both.

5. Breathe evenly and smoothly.

6. Hold the pose as long as you like. When you are ready to release, have your date help you up, holding your back and your hand.

Benefits: Increases flexibility in the back, legs, shoulders, arms, and spine.

To practice at home in a chair, slide your hips so they are on the edge of the seat. Lean backwards, placing the middle of your back on the seat edge and your hands on the floor, fingers facing you. Keep your forearms parallel. Breathe! When you come up, hold the sides of the chair. Bring your head up last.

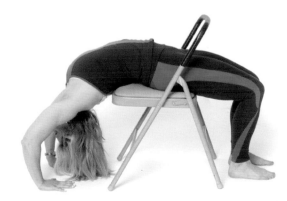

Happy Hour Hint

If there's some music playing, have your date lower you into this position as you're slow dancing. Simply have him dip you slowly and carefully onto the bar stool.

Ask Your Bartender for...

A Cosmopolitan, which is a cocktail made of vodka, triple sec, fresh lime, and a splash of cranberry juice. It is served in a martini glass, to accent its beauty.

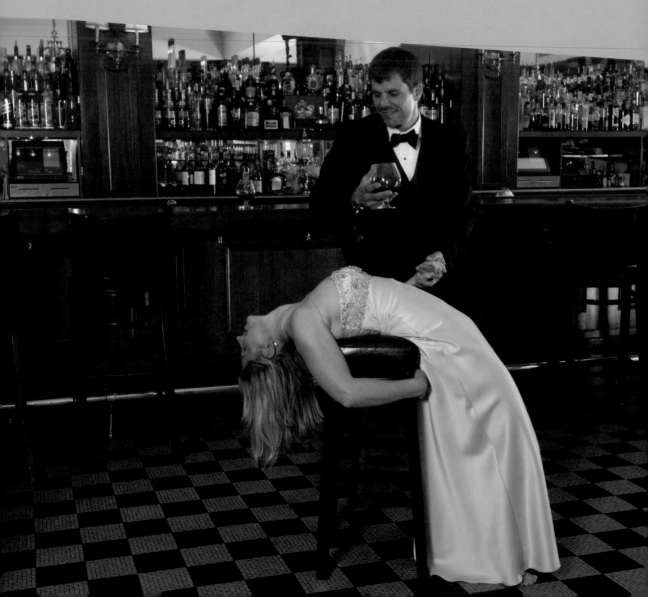

CHAPTER 7
HEAVEN FOR HANGOVERS

uch! Why did I drink so much last night? (Oh, yeah, now I remember.) Will this misery ever end?

Finally, an alternative to watching old movies all day until the torment diminishes. With a few simple yoga poses, your misery will give way to renewed tranquility, harmony, and more energy. And maybe even a sincere promise to practice more yoga.

RECIPE FOR RESTORED HARMONY:

1 PART PERSEVERANCE

1 PART FORGETTING OLD REMEDIES

2 PARTS TRUSTING YOUR BODY

GARNISH WITH A SMILE

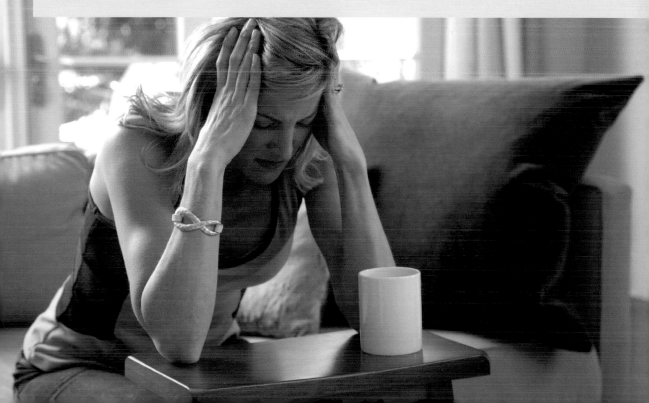

Post-Vodka Twist

Twisting poses are great to do when you have overindulged in the distilled spiritual realm. Twists help detoxify the liver and the bloodstream. In effect, twists wring the toxins out of the body. So be sure to drink a lot of water after you practice this segment.

WHAT YOU DO

1. Sit on the floor with your legs extended in front of you and a bar stool partially behind you and to your left.

2. Bend your right knee and place your right foot as close to your hips as possible. Bend your left leg and cross it over your right leg. Firmly press the sole of your left foot into the floor.

3. Make sure both hips are even on the floor. If one hip naturally rises, actively press it into the floor.

4. Place your hands on the rungs of a bar stool. With an inhalation, lift your spine. On an exhalation, twist from the very bottom of the spine toward the bar stool. Continue in this manner: On each inhalation, lengthen your spine. On each exhalation, twist a little more. Continue twisting deeper into the pose for 1 to 2 minutes.

5. Keep your face aligned with your chest.

6. Release on an exhalation, reverse your legs and the bar stool, and repeat on the other side.

Benefits: Detoxes the liver and bloodstream and increases flexibility and circulation in the vertebrae.

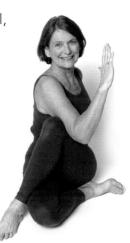

The difference between the bar stool pose and the traditional pose is this: Place the outside of your right upper arm on the outside of your left thigh. Press your arm and thigh against each other as you twist. Stay in the pose for 1 to 2 minutes. Then release with an exhalation, reverse your legs, and twist to the left for an equal amount of time.

Twists are good to practice because we must frequently twist in our everyday lives. Deliberate, active twisting—as we do in yoga—keeps us flexible in ways that stretching poses don't. Twists activate the spine, the surrounding muscles, and the internal organs. Twists improve circulation in the internal organs. Lengthening and stretching the spine through a practice of twists counteracts the negative effects of gravity, which compress the spine.

Ask Your Bartender For . . .

A Vodka Twist with citrus soda, cranberry juice . . . hold the vodka.

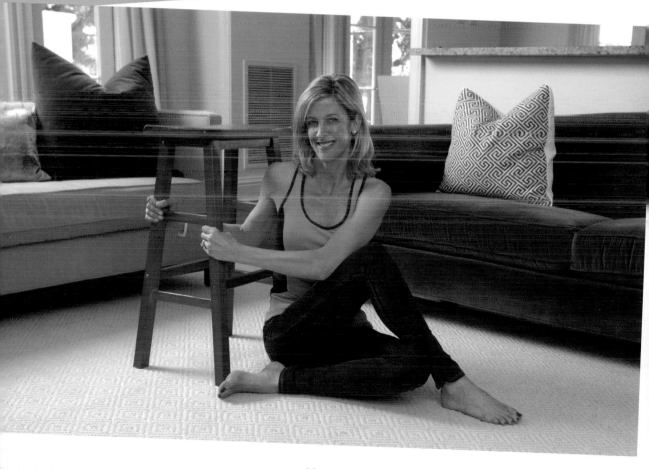

Twist, No Olive (and No Vodka)

Here's another twist to help release those toxins. This time it is Bharadvajasana, named for a great mythical warrior in ancient Hindu literature. You can definitely win the battle over your misery with this pose, which reduces back pain, enhances digestion, gives you a good stretch, and releases stress.

WHAT YOU DO

1. Sit with your legs extended in front of you and the bar stool on your right side.

2. Bend both legs and bring them close to your left hip. (If necessary, use your hand to get your feet closer to your hip.)

3. Place your left ankle on top of the arch of your right foot. Stretch your toes so they are as straight as possible.

4. Firmly press your hips into the floor.

5. Place your right hand slightly behind your right hip. Place your left hand on the bar stool.

6. On an inhalation, lift your spine. On an exhalation, twist toward the right. Twist from the very bottom of your spine.

7. Continue inhaling and lifting, exhaling and twisting a little deeper in the twist.

8. Gently unwind to release. Place the bar stool on your left side and repeat the pose, twisting to the left.

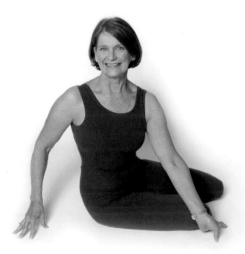

Benefits: This pose helps alleviate back pain and helps with digestion.

The traditional pose is performed with your hand on the outside of your thigh and your other hand slightly behind you to help you twist.

If one side of your hips keeps popping up, place a folded blanket beneath it and then press both hips down.

Ask Your Bartender For . . .

Sparkling water with a twist of lime.

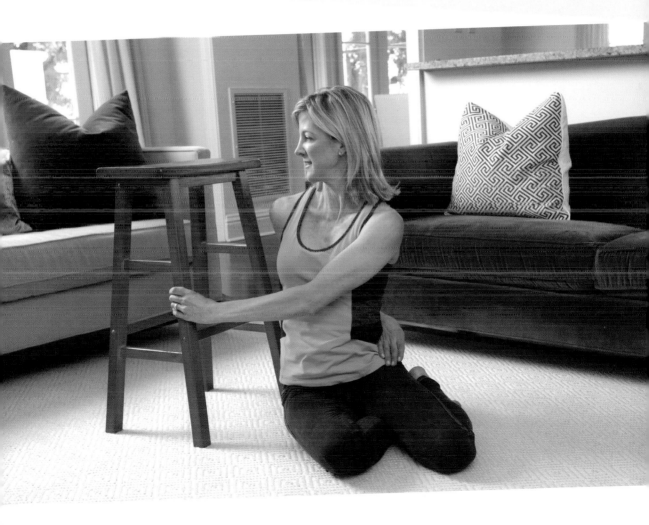

Death in the Afternoon

This pose may look a bit like the position you were in when you woke up after your last night of heavy libations. This is a passive variation of Standing Wide Angle pose, and naturally, you should not do this if you feel nauseated. If you feel bad, but not sick to your stomach, this pose will bring blood flow to your head, helping to relieve a headache and general achiness.

WHAT YOU DO

1. With your feet wide, lean over a bar stool with your front hip bones and lower abdomen on the stool.

2. Hold your elbows and completely drop your head.

3. Stay in the pose as long as you like. Release very slowly, and sit for a few moments so you do not get dizzy.

Benefits: Strengthens and stretches the inner back legs and spine, tones the abdominal organs, and calms the brain.

For the classic pose, stand with your feet approximately 4 feet wide, with your feet parallel and your toes pointing forward. Place your hands on your hips. From your hip crease, bend forward and place your hands to the floor. Extend your spine and keep your head in line with your spine.

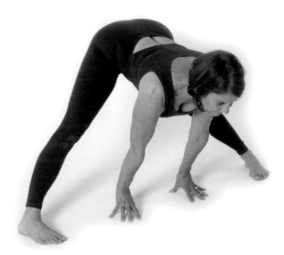

Happy Hour Hint

This pose will also release tension from your back, shoulders, and neck. You can do the passive version any time, particularly if you have lower back pain or your neck is aching.

Ask Your Bartender For . . .

Death in the Afternoon, which was aptly named—because if you have too many, you will want to die the next afternoon. This drink is also called the Hemingway or Hemingway Champagne, and it consists of absinthe and champagne. The cocktail, invented by Ernest Hemingway, shares a name with one of his books, *Death in the Afternoon*.

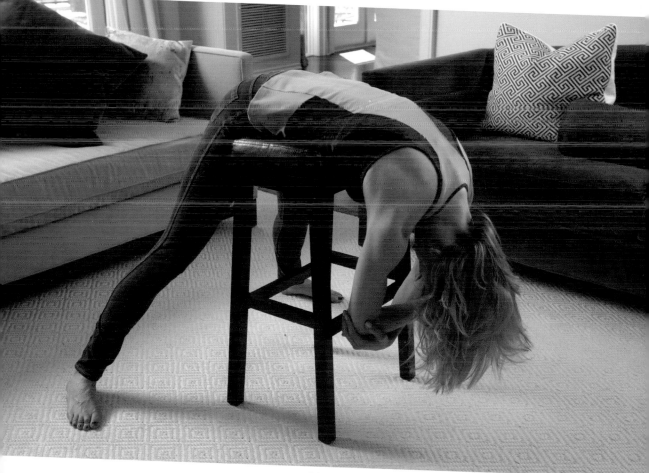

Corpse Reviver

If there is any pose that will revive you when you are hungover, it is Supported Plow pose. It completely restores you when you are tired, for any reason. It is a great headache cure, helps relieve sinus congestion and pain, and is a panacea for most common ailments. Try this pose rather than the Corpse Reviver cocktail.

WHAT YOU DO

1. Place the outside edge of a bolster about a foot from the couch or chair you will use to get started. Have the bar stool about 2 feet behind the bolster.

2. Lie down on the floor with your neck on the bolster.

3. Place your feet on the chair or sofa and lift your torso.

4. Place your hands on or near your shoulder blades. Adjust the top of your shoulders so they are completely on the prop, widening the tops of your shoulders.

5. Soften your throat and bring your chin toward your chest. When you are ready, using your hands to guide you, bring your legs over your head and place your feet, or the tops of your thighs, on the bar stool.

6. Stay in this pose as long as you like. You may even fall asleep in this pose. To release, bring your feet back to the sofa. Then bring your hips to the floor and rest with your legs on the sofa or chair for several minutes.

Benefits: This pose stretches the shoulders, improves digestion, and calms nerves.

For home practice, lie on the floor with your head facing the wall, with your shoulders on the bolster. Have one chair near your feet and another chair at the wall. Place the soles of your feet on the seat of the chair that is near your feet. Lift your torso, place your hands on your back to help you bring your legs up and over your head. Place your toes on the seat of the chair that is at the wall. Hold as long as you like. Release gently.

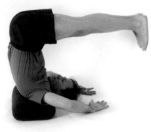
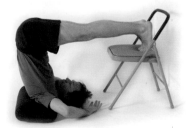

Getting into this pose can be a little tricky, so you may have to practice a few times before you get it right. Try experimenting with this pose before you really need it. You will be very happy that you practiced in advance because you will want to experience the healing effect it has on your body as often as needed.

Ask Your Bartender For . . .

The Corpse Reviver and Corpse Reviver 2, both which have been around at least since the 1930s. The original contains brandy, bitters, and crème de menthe, while the sequel has licorice liqueur, champagne, and lemon juice.

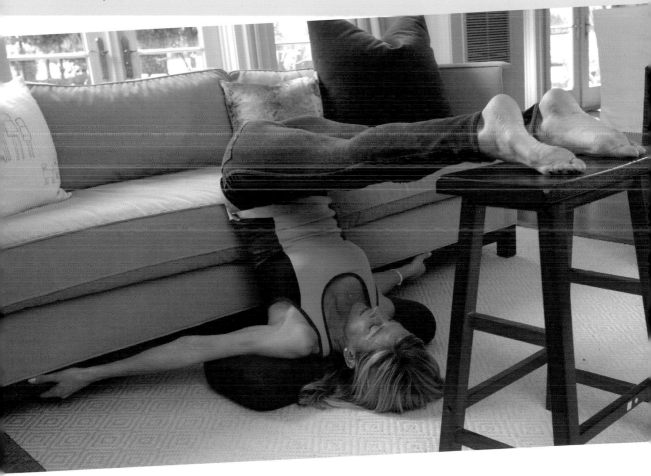

Sundowner Corpse

Here's another pose you might have done inadvertently after an evening of over imbibing. In Britain, a Sundowner is any alcoholic drink someone has at the end of the workday, which is usually at sundown. This version of the traditional Corpse pose can be done at the end of your Heaven for Hangovers series—or any day in lieu of the alcoholic sundowner.

WHAT YOU DO

1. Lie down on the floor and place your calves or your heels on a low bar stool.

2. Close your eyes and concentrate on your breathing. Start with normal breathing. After a few minutes, change your breathing rhythm by taking normal inhalations and long, slow, smooth exhalations. Use this rhythmic breathing for a few minutes and then return to normal breathing. You will probably fall asleep. Truly heavenly!

Benefits: Relieves back tension and releases anxiety. Very calming.

This pose differs from the traditional one in that you place your calves and/or feet on a low bar stool or on the seat of a chair, rather than having your legs stretched out on the floor. This is particularly good for those with back pain, as it allows the back muscles to relax and release more easily.

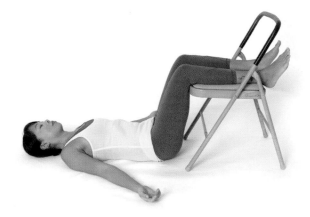

Happy Hour Hint

Before getting into the final pose, you may want to practice this a couple of times with different props, testing for maximum comfort and relaxation. Have some props handy: two blankets, a rolled hand towel, an eye cover, and maybe some earplugs. Lie down on the floor and place your feet on the seat of the bar stool or chair seat. If your head and neck are not completely comfortable, try a blanket or two under your head. If that isn't comfortable, try the rolled hand towel under your neck. Consider how comfortable that is. You may want to make the roll thinner or thicker by adding an extra towel. Once your head and neck are completely comfortable, place an eye cover (maybe a face towel) on your eyes, and earplugs in your ears. This way, you completely block out any disturbing noise and light.

Ask Your Bartender For . . .

A Sundowner, one recipe of which contains coconut rum, pineapple juice, and bitters.

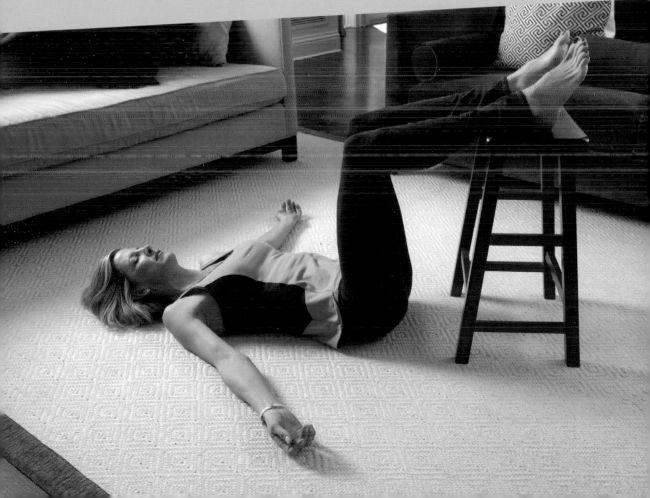

ACKNOWLEDGMENTS

My sincere gratitude to all those who have made this book the super fun project that it has been. First and foremost, Charlie Nurnberg, my publisher. Thank you, Charlie, for making *Bar Stool Yoga*, and two of my other books, great successes!

Great thanks to Steve Hunter, the fabulous photographer who, with his artistic eye and camera lens, captured the sheer joy that this book is. Some of his other photos can be seen on his website: www.fishbowlneworleans.com.

Thanks to my strikingly attractive models—you are the greatest!! The gorgeous ladies are: Dana Hammer, Syndey Gann, Cara Walton, Kristen Newman, Van Nguyen, Ananda Tinio, Jenna Wolf, Nancy Stechert, Trinh Do, Suzanne Even, and Mary Dawn Pugh. Those handsome guys pictured here are: Randy White, Bruno Prager, Mike Pugh, Jimmy "Salserito" McIvers, and Diem Do.

My uniquely kind and generous friend, Haiyan Khan, helped me with many aspects of the photo shoot. Haiyan did a little of everything: helping to set up the shots with his keen eye, helping the models align their poses, allowing us to use his yoga studio, even carrying equipment. Haiyan is a wonderfully compassionate person and a fantastic yoga teacher. Next time you are in New Orleans, take a class with Haiyan. You will be so happy in his class! http://haiyankhan.wix.com/swanriveryogaarabi.

The owners of the various bars and restaurants gave us the unique opportunity to photograph this fun book in "natural settings." *Martini Yoginis* and *Flirtini Night* were photographed at the world-famous Pat O'Brien's in the French Quarter of New Orleans. Visit this celebrated bar at www.patobriens.com and next time you are in New Orleans.

The legendary *Antoine's* restaurant, also in the French Quarter of New Orleans, graciously welcomed us to their *Hermes Bar* for *Puttin' on The Ritz*. Antoine's has been serving fabulous French-Creole food in a unique, French Quarter setting for almost 200 years. It is a "must have dinner there" destination. Check out their website: www.antoines.com.

Superior Grill and *Superior Seafood* owner, Bob Kirchoff, embraced this concept enthusiastically from the start. His iconic restaurants and bars on St. Charles Avenue in New Orleans are the settings for *Champagne and Oysters* and the cover photo. Check out their websites: www.superiorgrill.com and www.superiorseafoodnola.com.

With its unique, artsy atmosphere—and best coffee in the city—*Merchant Coffee and Wine Bar*, hosted us for *Too Many Tequila Sun(rise) Salutations.* Check out their coffee and their website, www.merchantneworleans.com.

And a special thanks to Trinh and Diem Do, who were models and opened their lovely home to us for *Shaken, Not Stirred* and *Heaven for Hangovers.*

Much gratitude to Cathy Robbins of *Belladonna Spa* for makeup artistry, commitment and enthusiasm for keeping us looking our best. You can reach her at www.belladonnaspa.com.

Great thanks to my husband, Van, who—once again—has enthusiastically given his love, joy, and support to me while I have "abandoned" him to work on another book.

And, to my nephew, Blake. Thank you, Blake, for keeping me entertained and stress-free with your charm, humor, and many hours of fun and games when I was not on location.

INDEX